T5-APB-784

Clinical Pocket Manual™

Emergency Care

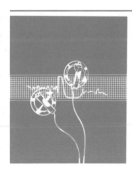

NURSING85 BOOKS™
SPRINGHOUSE CORPORATION
SPRINGHOUSE, PENNSYLVANIA

Clinical Pocket Manual™ Series

PROGRAM DIRECTOR
Jean Robinson

CLINICAL DIRECTOR
Barbara McVan, RN

ART DIRECTOR
John Hubbard

EDITORIAL MANAGER
Susan R. Williams

EDITORS
Lisa Z. Cohen
Kathy E. Goldberg
Virginia P. Peck

CLINICAL EDITORS
Joan E. Mason, RN, EdM
Diane Schweisguth, RN, BSN

COPY SUPERVISOR
David R. Moreau

DESIGNER
Maria Errico

PRODUCTION COORDINATOR
Susan Powell-Mishler

Material in this book was adapted from the following series: Nurse's Reference Library, Nursing photobook, New Nursing Skillbook, NursingNow, and Nurse's Clinical Library.

CPM2-011085

Library of Congress Cataloging-in-Publication Data

Main entry under title:

Emergency care.

(Clinical pocket manual)
"Nursing85 books."
Includes index.
1. Emergency nursing—Handbooks, manuals, etc.
2. Emergency medicine—Handbooks, manuals, etc. I. Springhouse Corporation. II. Series.
RT120.E4E426 1985 616'.025 85-12706
ISBN 0-87434-004-7

CONTENTS

Nursing85 Books™

CLINICAL POCKET MANUAL™ SERIES
Diagnostic Tests
Emergency Care
Fluids and Electrolytes
Signs and Symptoms
Cardiovascular Care
Respiratory Care
Critical Care
Neurologic Care

NURSING NOW™ SERIES
Shock
Hypertension
Drug Interactions
Cardiac Crises
Respiratory Emergencies
Pain

NURSE'S CLINICAL LIBRARY™
Cardiovascular Disorders
Respiratory Disorders
Endocrine Disorders
Neurologic Disorders
Renal and Urologic Disorders
Gastrointestinal Disorders
Neoplastic Disorders
Immune Disorders

NURSING PHOTOBOOK™ SERIES
Providing Respiratory Care
Managing I.V. Therapy
Dealing with Emergencies
Giving Medications
Assessing Your Patients
Using Monitors
Providing Early Mobility
Giving Cardiac Care
Performing GI Procedures
Implementing Urologic Procedures
Controlling Infection
Ensuring Intensive Care
Coping with Neurologic Disorders
Caring for Surgical Patients
Working with Orthopedic Patients
Nursing Pediatric Patients
Helping Geriatric Patients
Attending Ob/Gyn Patients
Aiding Ambulatory Patients
Carrying Out Special Procedures

NURSE'S REFERENCE LIBRARY®
Diseases
Diagnostics
Drugs
Assessment
Procedures
Definitions
Practices
Emergencies
Signs and Symptoms

NURSE REVIEW™ SERIES
Cardiac Problems
Respiratory Problems

Nursing85 DRUG HANDBOOK™

The 90-Second Assessment

In an emergency, follow the ABCs of assessment to establish the priorities of your nursing care.

AIRWAY

Check the patient's airway for signs of obstruction: wheezing, stridor, or choking. If he makes a violent effort to sit up, let him do so. This may be a reflex action to establish an open airway.

Priorities:
• Position the patient on his back. Carefully straighten his arms and legs.
• Use the head-tilt–neck-lift or head-tilt-chin-lift maneuver to raise the tongue away from the back of the throat. This may be enough to start the patient breathing.
　Caution: When you suspect neck injury, don't use the head-tilt–neck-lift maneuver, but attempt to open the airway with a modified jaw-thrust.
• To relieve airway obstruction: insert oral or nasal airway, then suction patient. If patient is comatose, insert an endotracheal tube.

BREATHING

Check the patient's breathing to determine if his respirations are adequate. Look, listen, and feel for signs of breathing by placing your ear close to his mouth and nose to detect air movement. Watch his chest and abdomen to see if they rise and fall.

Priorities:
• Auscultate breath sounds bilaterally.
• If the patient hasn't started breathing spontaneously after you've performed the head-tilt or jaw-thrust maneuver, ventilate him immediately using the mouth-to-mouth or mouth-to-nose technique.
　Nursing tip: If the patient has a stoma from a tracheostomy, give mouth-to-stoma ventilations.
　You may also relieve respiratory insufficiency with oxygen or positive-pressure ventilation.
Continued

EMERGENCY BASICS

The 90-Second Assessment
Continued

CIRCULATION

Check the patient's circulation by feeling for a pulse in the carotid artery. If the neck's been injured, feel instead for a femoral pulse. If no pulse exists, the patient's circulation has stopped.

Priorities:
• Perform closed-chest massage if circulation has stopped.
• Control external hemorrhage by applying direct pressure over the bleeding site.

• Control shock by administering I.V. fluids. Insert Foley catheter to measure output and assess fluid replacement. Measure vital signs and insert CVP line to monitor effectiveness of fluid replacement. Order arterial blood gas studies, complete blood count (CBC), blood urea nitrogen (BUN), glucose, and electrolytes to establish baseline values and monitor effectiveness of therapy.

Special Consideration

"I think I'm gonna die." You've probably heard this and similar statements many times, from patients with many different disorders. But how often do you take such a patient seriously?

Rather than being a cry for extra attention, a statement like this may be a valuable clue to your patient's condition—a clue that only he can provide. For example, a keen sense of impending doom often accompanies the persistent chest pain that precedes a myocardial infarction.

So *listen* to your patient, and take any statement he makes about his condition as a signal to assess him extra carefully. Don't let his premonitions become reality.

Body-System Emergency Assessment Checklist

VITAL SIGNS

What to assess:
● Auscultate or palpate the patient's blood pressure.
● Note the rate, depth, pattern, and symmetry of his respirations.
● Palpate his radial pulse and note its rate, rhythm, and strength.
● Take his temperature.

GENERAL SURVEY

What to assess:
● Observe the patient's level of consciousness, behavior, and mental status.
● Inspect his body for obvious deformities due to trauma.
● Observe him for severe, moderate, or mild distress and anxiety.
● Inspect his skin for color, moisture, turgor, temperature, and ecchymoses.
● Note the presence of any distinctive odors on his breath, such as alcohol or acetone.
● Note his degree of mobility.

NEUROLOGIC

What to assess:
● Determine the patient's level of consciousness.
● Inspect his pupils for size, symmetry, and reaction to light.
● Observe him for abnormal posture (decorticate or decerebrate).
● Inspect and palpate his scalp for trauma or deformities.
● Assess the sensory and motor responses of each affected body part.
● Observe him for facial asymmetry, and listen for slurred speech.
● Assess deep tendon reflexes.

EYES, EARS, NOSE, AND THROAT

What to assess:
● Inspect the patient's eyes for burns.
● Inspect and palpate his face and his eyes, ears, nose, and throat for trauma or deformities.
● Assess his speech for dysphonia or aphonia.
● Inspect his ears and nose for bleeding, drainage, and foreign objects.
● Inspect his oral mucosa for color, hydration, inflammation, and bleeding.
● Inspect and palpate his thyroid gland for tenderness and enlargement.
● Inspect his oropharynx for signs of burns due to ingestion of caustic agents.
● Assess his gross visual acuity and eye movements.

Continued

Body-System Emergency Assessment Checklist
Continued

RESPIRATORY

What to assess:
• Observe the patient for use of accessory muscles, for paradoxical chest movements, and for respiratory distress.
• Inspect his chest for contour, symmetry, and deformities or trauma.
• Auscultate his lungs for adventitious sounds and increased or decreased breath sounds.
• Palpate his chest for tenderness, pain, and crepitation.

CARDIOVASCULAR

What to assess:
• Palpate the patient's peripheral pulses—especially of each affected body part—for rate, rhythm, quality, and symmetry.
• Inspect him for jugular vein distention.
• Inspect and palpate his extremities for edema, mottling and cyanosis, and temperature change.
• Auscultate his heart sounds for timing, intensity, pitch, and quality, and note the presence of murmurs, rubs, or extra sounds.
• Auscultate blood pressure in both arms.

GASTROINTESTINAL

What to assess:
• Inspect the patient's abdomen for obvious signs of trauma.
• Inspect any vomitus or stool for amount, color, presence of blood, and consistency.
• Inspect his abdomen for distention.
• Auscultate his abdomen for bowel sounds.
• Palpate his abdomen for pain, tenderness, or rigidity.
• Percuss his abdomen for possible ascites.

GENITOURINARY

What to assess:
• Inspect the patient's external genitalia for bleeding, ecchymoses, edema, or hematoma.
• Palpate his abdomen for suprapubic pain.
• Palpate his external genitalia for pain or tenderness.
• Palpate for costovertebral angle (CVA) tenderness.

Continued

Body-System Emergency Assessment Checklist
Continued

MUSCULOSKELETAL

What to assess:
• Inspect the patient's body for trauma and deformities.
• Gently palpate his cervical spine for tenderness and deformities.
• Palpate his vertebral spine and percuss his costovertebral areas for tenderness.
• Inspect his skin for color, ecchymoses, pigmentation, and discoloration.

• Palpate his pulses distal to any injury.
• Palpate his area of suspected injury for tenderness, pain, and edema.
• Assess his motor and sensory responses.
• Observe the range of motion of his injured extremity.
• Inspect his skin for needle marks.
• Assess for nuchal rigidity.

Quantifying Pain

As a nurse, you know that quantifying pain is very difficult because what's excruciating for one patient may be merely uncomfortable for another. Of course, this happens because everyone's pain threshold is different.

Here's a tip for obtaining an accurate baseline assessment of your patient's pain: Try asking him to rate his pain on a scale of 1 to 10, 1 representing no pain and 10 representing the worst pain he's ever felt. This technique gives your patient a way of measuring and expressing his

pain. It also involves him actively in the assessment, which may have the added benefit of helping to reduce his anxiety.

You may also use a linear scale with the words: no pain, mild pain, moderate pain, severe pain, or unbearable pain. The patient selects the word that best represents his pain intensity. Although everyone interprets pain differently, this scale can be administered quickly and interpreted easily. Both scales provide baseline data that you can use when you assess his pain again.

Advanced Life Support

Advanced life support (ALS) measures support cardiopulmonary resuscitation (CPR) by treating the physical changes and complications that can occur after cardiac arrest. These measures include the use of special techniques and equipment to help establish and maintain ventilation and circulation, the use of cardiac monitors to detect abnormal heart rate and rhythm, the insertion of a peripheral I.V. line, drug therapy, cardiac defibrillation, and the insertion of an artificial pacemaker. When the patient's condition stabilizes, the cause of cardiac arrest can be treated. Many ALS techniques, including defibrillation and drug administration, can be initiated by a specially trained nurse under standing orders; some techniques may be performed only by a doctor.

The techniques and equipment used in ALS depend on the patient's needs and on the setting. Usually, the following sequence of ALS procedures is required:

• First, alert co-workers and obtain a crash cart, which usually contains all equipment necessary for ALS.
• Because CPR requires a firm surface to be effective, place a cardiac arrest board or other flat, rigid support under the patient's back. Start CPR immediately *to ensure oxygenation and perfusion of vital organs.* Continue CPR while other ALS equipment is being set up. During later ALS procedures, avoid interrupting CPR for longer than 15 seconds.
• Set up the EKG machine *to monitor cardiovascular status continuously and to help determine proper therapy.* Because the EKG doesn't indicate the effectiveness of cardiac compression, take central (carotid or femoral) pulses frequently.
• Attempt to obtain a medical history from the patient's family or companion *to learn the probable cause of the arrest and to determine contraindications for resuscitation.*
• Insert a peripheral I.V. line for fluid and emergency drug administration. Use a large blood vessel, such as the brachial vein, *because smaller peripheral vessels tend to collapse quickly during arrest.* Use a large-gauge needle *to prevent dislodgment or injury to the vein, with extravasation and vessel collapse.* Use dextrose 5% in water to start the infusion; other fluids, such as normal saline solution, counteract circulatory collapse caused by hypovolemia and may be ordered as appropriate later.

Continued

Advanced Life Support
Continued

• Perform defibrillation and administer appropriate drugs, such as epinephrine, isoproterenol, and calcium chloride, which stimulate cardiac pacemaker discharge. These drugs treat asystole without defibrillation but can cause dysrhythmias, such as ventricular fibrillation, which require defibrillation. (Although cardiac monitoring should be started before defibrillation, a single countershock delivered to the heart without monitoring isn't harmful, and immediate "blind" defibrillation may prove lifesaving; however, blind defibrillation of children is not recommended.

• If the patient fails to respond quickly to CPR, a single countershock, and basic drug therapy, insert a ventilatory device, such as an endotracheal tube or oxygen cannula. After the device is in place, discontinue mouth-to-mouth breathing, but maintain respiratory assistance with an Ambu bag. Oxygen is used jointly with most of these devices.

• Remove oral secretions with portable or wall suction, and insert a nasogastric tube *to relieve or prevent gastric distention.*

• If the patient responds to the preceding treatments and has severe bradycardia, with reduced cardiac output (as in acute heart block),

vasopressors may be given. If these do not sufficiently raise heart rate and cardiac output, the doctor may insert a temporary cardiac pacemaker to boost the heart's faltering electrical activity to a near-normal rate.

• In most cases, when the patient's condition begins to stabilize or when preliminary ALS steps have been taken, he may be transported to a special-care area. If necessary, use a circulatory assist device, such as a manual or automatic chest compressor, *to provide external cardiac compression during transport.* Because the device compresses the sternum 1½" to 2" (3.8 to 5 cm), position the patient carefully *to avoid accidental compression of the ribs or epigastric area, resulting in rib fracture and possible liver laceration.*

• Begin direct therapy as ordered *to treat the underlying cause of the patient's arrest.* For example, if arrest resulted from an acute hypovolemic crisis, replace blood volume and apply Medical Antishock Trousers (MAST) *to redirect circulating blood from the extremities into the central circulation.* Or use acute dialysis to clear endogenous or exogenous toxins that may have caused the arrest.

EMERGENCY BASICS

Using Accident Information to Predict Injuries

When you're assessing an accident victim, every second counts. You simply don't have time to do a complete head-to-toe assessment and to obtain a detailed health history. So how can you make the most of every second? As quickly as you can, find out what type of accident caused the damage. Then, knowing that each major type of accident has a distinctive mechanism of injury, you can predict the types of injuries your patient's likely to have and focus your assessment accordingly.

This chart shows you the mechanisms of injury and related possible injuries for major types of accidents and for assaults.

TYPE	MECHANISM OF INJURY	POSSIBLE INJURIES
MOTOR VEHICLE COLLISIONS (OCCUPANT INJURIES)		
Head-on	• Body travels down and under, striking knees on dashboard, then chest on steering wheel	• Knee dislocation, femur fracture, posterior fracture or dislocation of hip, cardiac contusion, aortic tears and dissection
	• Body travels up and over, snapping head forward (hitting windshield) and striking lower chest or upper abdomen on steering wheel	• Head trauma, hyperflexion or hyperextension, cervical spine injuries, rib fractures, intraabdominal injuries
Rear-end	• Body travels forward as head remains in place, then snaps back across backrest or headrest	• Whiplash injuries of third to fourth cervical vertebrae
	• If frontal impact's also involved, body travels forward and hits dashboard and steering wheel	• Injuries from frontal impact (such as cardiac contusion, rib fractures, intraabdominal injuries, intrathoracic injuries)

Continued

Using Accident Information to Predict Injuries
Continued

TYPE	MECHANISM OF INJURY	POSSIBLE INJURIES

MOTOR VEHICLE COLLISIONS (OCCUPANT INJURIES)

TYPE	MECHANISM OF INJURY	POSSIBLE INJURIES
Lateral impact	• Body slams into door, injuring chest, pelvis, and neck	• Chest injuries with or without humerus fracture, pelvic or femur fractures, contralateral neck injuries (tears or sprain of neck ligaments)
Rotational force	• Body reacts to collision as vehicle hits stationary object and rotates around it	• Combination of head-on and lateral impact collision injuries
Rollover	• Body stays in place (if restrained) or bounces around as vehicle rolls over	• Various collision injuries, similar to rotational-force injuries
Seat belt	• Body compresses against lap belt worn too high (above anterior superior iliac spine)	• Abdominal organ injuries, thoracic or lumbar spine injuries
	• Body compresses against shoulder belt	• Shoulder and neck injuries

MOTOR VEHICLE ACCIDENTS (PEDESTRIAN INJURIES)

TYPE	MECHANISM OF INJURY	POSSIBLE INJURIES
Head-on (Waddell's triad)	• Body impacts with bumper and hood	• Femur and chest injuries

Continued

EMERGENCY BASICS

Using Accident Information to Predict Injuries
Continued

TYPE	MECHANISM OF INJURY	POSSIBLE INJURIES

MOTOR VEHICLE ACCIDENTS (PEDESTRIAN INJURIES)

TYPE	MECHANISM OF INJURY	POSSIBLE INJURIES
Head-on *Continued*	• Force propels victim toward third point of impact (when body comes to rest)	• At third point of impact, contralateral skull injuries
Lateral impact	• Lower and upper leg impact with bumper and hood	• Tibia, fibula, and femur fractures • Ligament damage in opposite knee because of excess stress

MOTORCYCLE COLLISIONS

TYPE	MECHANISM OF INJURY	POSSIBLE INJURIES
Head-on	• Body (head and chest) strikes handlebars	• Head, chest, and abdominal injuries, bilateral femur fractures
Angular	• Motorcycle falls on body	• Crush injuries to lower limbs, open fractures
Ejection	• Body is thrown from motorcycle into an object	• Head and spine injuries, deceleration injuries

ASSAULTS

TYPE	MECHANISM OF INJURY	POSSIBLE INJURIES
Beating	• Body—especially head, neck, abdomen— is struck by blunt object or fist	• Soft tissue injuries, major organ injuries in specific area of blunt trauma

Continued

Using Accident Information to Predict Injuries
Continued

TYPE	MECHANISM OF INJURY	POSSIBLE INJURIES

ASSAULTS

Stab wound	• Body—usually chest or abdomen—is stabbed with sharp weapon	• Blood loss, sucking chest wound, organ penetration, heart or major vessel penetration (direction of attack, type of weapon, and attacker's strength determine severity)
Missile injuries	• Projectile from a pistol, rifle, shotgun, or explosion enters and exits body, or enters and lodges in body • Projectile follows path of least resistance	• Range from minor puncture to life-threatening wound of chest, abdomen, or head • Lacerated tissue in bullet's path, possible injury to remote organs
	• Projectile forms cavity as it releases energy into tissues in its path • Energy travels through affected tissues and injures other tissues • Close contact may cause muzzle blast injury	• Initial wound, subsequent tissue injury (not necessarily in direct path of bullet), secondary infection • Internal tissue and bone damage • Internal tissue and bone damage

JUMPS AND FALLS

Compression force	• Person falls from a height and lands on his heels	• Bilateral fractures of calcaneus

Continued

Using Accident Information to Predict Injuries
Continued

TYPE	MECHANISM OF INJURY	POSSIBLE INJURIES
JUMPS AND FALLS		
Compression force Continued	• Forward momentum causes acute flexion of lumbar spine, then continued forward momentum causes person to land on outstretched hands	• Compression fractures of vertebrae • Colles' fracture of wrists
Indirect force	• Person falls backward and lands on back and head	• Spine and head injuries, tibia and fibula fractures
Twisting force	• Person falls (usually during sports activity) and twists legs	• Tibia and fibula fractures

Special Consideration

Secondary injuries: If your patient has a *penetrating injury,* you can commonly expect less secondary trauma than if he has a blunt injury because a penetrating injury usually involves less energy. Stab wounds in particular are relatively low-energy wounds that may involve only one or two body systems.

If your patient has a *blunt injury,* you may have difficulty determining which organs are injured and whether he has secondary injuries. This is because blunt trauma involves indirect as well as direct forces, so it may cause injuries at some distance from the site where the major force was applied.

When Your Patient Can't Communicate

The best way to get information about your patient with an emergency, of course, is for *him* to tell you about his history and what happened to him. But suppose your patient can't talk—for example, what if he's unconscious? Here are some suggested ways to get the emergency assessment information you need:

• Question anyone who may be able to provide information—for example, family members or friends, witnesses, or rescue personnel.

• Is the patient wearing a Medic Alert bracelet (or necklace)? Be sure to check for this and—if he's wearing one—to note what it says about his medical status.

• Has he been transferred from a nursing home, outpatient clinic, or referral agency? Call them for information.

• Does he have any prescription medications with him? If he does, call the pharmacy listed on the bottle. Most pharmacies keep patient profile cards containing significant medical information, including other medications their customers may be taking.

• What is the medication? It may indicate a preexisting condition. For example, if he's taking procainamide hydrochloride (Pronestyl), you know he's probably had prior episodes of cardiac dysrhythmias.

• Who is his doctor? Is the name on a medication bottle? If it is, call the doctor for more information. Is the doctor a cardiologist, a neurosurgeon, a psychiatrist? The answer will help you define your patient's problem or illness.

• Has he been in your hospital before? You may be able to locate the old chart or ED record.

Being a Good Samaritan: Some Do's and Don'ts

DO's

- Care for the victim in the vehicle if you can do so safely.
- Move him if he's in danger and if conditions at the scene permit.
- Keep the victim's airway patent.
- Stop his bleeding.
- Keep him warm.
- Determine his level of consciousness.
- Determine the possibility of fractures.
- Ask him where he feels pain.

DON'Ts

- Don't move the victim needlessly.
- Don't try to straighten his arms and legs.
- Don't carry him or force him to walk.
- Don't speculate about who's the guilty party in the accident.
- Don't allow unskilled personnel to attend or treat the victim.
- Don't leave the scene until *skilled* personnel arrive to assume care of the victim.
- Don't give the injured person's personal property to anyone except the police or family members.

Sample Good Samaritan Act

Almost every state and Canadian province has its own Good Samaritan act. All of the acts, however, are basically like the one reprinted in part here, from the state of Florida.

(1) This act shall be known and cited as the "Good Samaritan Act."

(2) Any person, including those licensed to practice medicine, who gratuitously and in good faith renders emergency care or treatment at the scene of an emergency outside of a hospital, doctor's office, or other place having proper medical equipment, without objection of the injured victim or victims thereof, shall not be held liable for any civil damages as a result of such care or treatment or as a result of any act or failure to act in providing or arranging further medical treatment where the person acts as an ordinary reasonably prudent man would have acted under the same or similar circumstances.

Can Your Patient Refuse Lifesaving Treatment?

A court will usually allow a patient to refuse treatment if he can make a sound decision. Or, if the patient's a child, typically his parents may decide on his care. But courts will intervene sometimes when a patient or parent refuses lifesaving treatment. Here are some court cases showing how courts have handled such situations:

• In *Collins v. David* (1964), the court overruled a wife's refusal of surgery for her unconscious husband, even though such a refusal is frequently ruled valid.

• A court may view a patient's responsibility for a child as reason to overrule the patient's refusal of lifesaving treatment. In *Application of the President and Directors of Georgetown College, Inc.* (1964), the court ordered a blood transfusion for a Jehovah's Witness, mother of an infant, who refused to consent to the transfusion.

• If a patient's pregnant and refuses lifesaving treatment so that her child's life is also endangered, a court may reverse the patient's decision. In *Jefferson v. Griffin Spalding County Hospital Authority* (1981), a pregnant woman with a complete placenta previa, who had refused to consent to a cesarean section, was denied the right to refuse the surgery. The court gave custody of her unborn child to a state agency, which then had full authority to consent to the surgery.

• The courts will not normally permit a child's parent or legal guardian to refuse consent for treatment that will save the child's life. *In re Sampson* (1972) was such a case.

Besides its concern for preserving a patient's life or protecting his dependents, a state may ask a court to prevent a patient's irrational self-destruction, to preserve the ethical integrity of health-care providers, or to protect public health. You should know, however, that each such case must be decided separately. Courts don't always rule that the state's interest overrides the patient's rights under common law and the U.S. Constitution.

Handling Evidence Properly

When police ask you to obtain evidence or to take charge of it in the ED, follow these general guidelines for identifying and preserving it:

• Identify and label *each piece* of evidence.

• Give the patient a receipt for *all* personal property taken from him. Be sure the hospital keeps a copy of this receipt.

• Preserve the evidence in its original state as much as possible—by taking steps to protect it while handling it as little as possible.

• Maintain the necessary "chain of custody" over the evidence, while it's in your custody, by obtaining the signature of each person who handles it. When *you* relinquish custody of the evidence, be sure to obtain a receipt for it.

• Protect a rape victim's legal rights by ensuring that all specimens are carefully labeled and that transfer of the evidence from the nurse or doctor to the police is carefully documented.

Q Am I covered by the Good Samaritan act if I respond to an emergency outside the hospital while I'm on duty?

A That depends on two things: the wording of the act in your state and court decisions, if any, that interpret that act.

Q If a doctor and I respond to the same emergency, does the Good Samaritan act provide us with the same coverage?

A Not necessarily. In some states, the Good Samaritan act for nurses is completely different from the Good Samaritan act for doctors. Contact your state's board of nursing to find out what's true for your state.

Recognizing Child Abuse

Whenever an injured child is brought to the ED, be sure to assess him for possible abuse. Remember, too, that the law requires reporting of all incidents of suspected child abuse to designated authorities.

Assessment:

Your assessment of an injured child should always include an evaluation of:
- his injuries
- his general appearance
- his behavior and the behavior of whoever accompanies him.

First, carefully assess the child's injuries. Suspect child abuse if you see:
- multiple bruises, abrasions, or lacerations
- fractures (especially Salter type II or "bucket handle" fractures, or rib fractures)
- burns from immersion in very hot water or from cigarettes; branding appearance of burns
- head trauma, facial injuries, or retinal hemorrhage
- internal injuries
- signs of genital or rectal trauma—discharges, bruises, or lacerations.

Note the location of burns, bruises, and lacerations; on an abused child, common areas for these injuries include the cheeks, trunk, genitals, buttocks, thighs, and arms.

Note the child's general appearance. An abused child is likely to come to the hospital dressed inappropriately for the weather, and he may have a dirty, unkempt appearance. He's likely to be shorter and to weigh less than the average for his age. And he may have several cuts and bruises, in various stages of healing, or unusual skin markings or scars. If he's been beaten, these markings may be in the shape of the object used, such as an electrical cord, a hand, a wire hanger, a coiled rope, or a broad strap or belt.

Observe the child's behavior. An abused child is likely to
- be underactive or hyperactive
- have a blank look
- seem especially fearful of his parents or cling to them in terror
- be extremely passive or drowsy or display other erratic or inappropriate behavior, indicating possible drug intoxication
- move away when you try to touch him.

Finally, note the parents' behavior, if they're the ones who've brought the child for treatment. Abusive parents are frequently uncooperative. They may hesitate or refuse to give you any information, refuse to give consent for diagnostic studies, or try to remove the child from the hospital before you can do a thorough examination. They may demand instant

Continued

Recognizing Child Abuse
Continued

treatment, complain about their own problems and other problems unrelated to the child's injury, and generally overreact or underreact to the seriousness of the situation.

Some abusive parents may react inappropriately by appearing totally uninterested in their child's problem; by giving you a history that doesn't explain the child's injury; by presenting contradictory or inconsistent versions of the injury-causing incident to different hospital personnel; or by blaming a third party, such as a sibling or neighbor, for the child's injury.

Other abusive parents will admit that they caused their child's injuries, yet defend their actions as justified punishment for the child's behavior.

When you talk to the parents, use a nonjudgmental approach, and focus on their concerns rather than on their child's.

Remember, you don't know *for sure* that they've abused their child, no matter how strong your suspicions are. Keep in mind that parents may be indirectly asking for help when they voice insistent complaints or bring their child's injuries to attention.

Documenting and reporting:
If your assessment findings lead you to suspect that the child's a victim of abuse, inform the doctor on duty of your suspicions. Expect him to order total body X-rays, a blood coagulation profile, and toxicology studies of the child's blood and urine.

If you continue to suspect child abuse after receiving the test results and talking with the parents, follow your hospital's protocol for notifying the appropriate state agency. (Many states impose a criminal penalty for failure to report.) State laws vary, so be sure you're familiar with the laws of your state.

Help the doctor explain to the parents that their child's history and physical findings cause you to suspect abuse and that you must report your suspicions. If they become alarmed, explain that you're making the report because the law requires it. Maintain a nonjudgmental attitude.

Finally, document all your findings carefully, completely, and objectively. Include the information you've gathered, the information you've given to the parents, and your subsequent actions, such as reporting the incident. Remember that in a court hearing, deciding factors could include your description of the child's injuries, the information you obtain from his parents, and your impressions of the parent-child interaction.

Consent to Photograph an Abused Child

You're on duty in your hospital's ED when a social worker brings in a girl, age 6, who's a possible victim of child abuse. The social worker asks you to photograph the girl's injuries to document them.

Can you legally take photographs of the patient?

No, but you can arrange for it. In most states, either an agency caseworker or the local police can photograph child abuse injuries without parental consent. In states that don't specifically grant the right to photograph, the examining doctor has the responsibility to authorize photographs, because the duty to report implies a responsibility to preserve any evidence. If the parents are present and object to photographs, the doctor should contact law enforcement officials to secure a court order.

All 50 states now have laws requiring that doctors and social workers (among other professionals) report suspected child abuse in children under age 16 or 18, depending on the state. These laws also offer professional care givers some immunity from liability, as long as they act in good faith.

Some states have designated reporting agencies. These agencies have 24-hour-a-day coverage and will send a caseworker to investigate night or day. Find out the appropriate agency you should contact when you suspect child abuse, and post the number near the ED telephone.

Child abuse reporting laws are far from standardized, so ED personnel should request a specific procedure from the hospital administration. Obviously, the administration should design a procedure that meets all state reporting laws.

Hidden Threat: Occult Bleeding

With multiple-trauma patients, you must be alert to signs of occult bleeding. This illustration shows the usual sites of such bleeding, along with the probable causes.

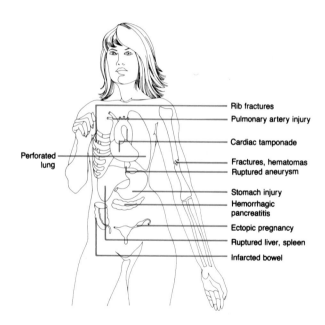

Rib fractures
Pulmonary artery injury

Cardiac tamponade

Perforated lung

Fractures, hematomas
Ruptured aneurysm

Stomach injury
Hemorrhagic pancreatitis

Ectopic pregnancy

Ruptured liver, spleen

Infarcted bowel

Priorities for Managing Musculoskeletal Injuries in Multiple-Trauma Patients

A patient with multiple trauma presents a real challenge to your nursing skills. His injuries are so serious, he'll require several doctors and nurses to stabilize several body systems simultaneously. Here's what you need to know about prioritizing his *musculoskeletal injuries* once you've:

• assessed and stabilized his ABCs

• applied a cervical collar to immobilize his head and neck

• inserted an I.V. for fluid and medication administration

• performed a rapid head-to-toe physical examination, paying particular attention to deformities, mobility of extremities, and abnormal swelling. The data from this examination guide your setting of priorities for managing the patient's multiple injuries.

With injuries in *any* body system, the rule is always *to care for the most life-threatening injuries first.* For musculoskeletal injuries in multiple trauma patients, you'll generally prioritize your emergency assessment and intervention in this manner:
1. cervical spine
2. chest
3. pelvis
4. skull
5. abdomen
6. extremities.

Of course, you'll change this order if a lesser injury becomes life-threatening, such as a bone fracture that causes obvious cardiopulmonary compromise or neurovascular impairment. You'll also change priorities if the patient has a distended abdomen and decreased blood pressure, indicating life-threatening occult abdominal hemorrhage.

And remember: sometimes an obvious injury—an open fracture, for example—may *look* dangerous, but it may not be nearly as life-threatening as a closed fracture that's causing internal hemorrhage.

Use the following chart as a guideline for prioritizing your multiple-trauma patient's musculoskeletal injuries.

Continued

EMERGENCY BASICS

Priorities for Managing Musculoskeletal Injuries in Multiple-Trauma Patients
Continued

PRIORITY 1
Prepare the patient for X-rays of his:
• lateral cervical spine
• chest (upright, if possible)
• pelvis, including a cystogram if he has hematuria. Check for occult fractures not found by physical examination.

If these X-rays show fractures, *intervene* as ordered. Expect to provide massive blood replacement and to assist with external skeletal fixation and laparotomy if life-threatening occult bleeding is also present.

PRIORITY 2
Immobilize fractures or dislocations in this order:
• bones causing occult hemorrhage, such as the pelvis
• bones causing neurovascular impairment, such as posterior dislocation of the hip
• large bones with obvious fractures, such as the femur or humerus
• smaller bones with obvious fractures, such as the ulna.

PRIORITY 3
Prepare the patient for X-ray of his:
• skull
• abdomen
• extremities. *Intervene* as ordered if injuries are found in these X-rays. Close lacerations and dress wounds.

PRIORITY 4
Prepare the patient for further studies, as indicated:
• CT scan
• IVP
• additional X-rays
• surgery
• ICU monitoring.

Special Consideration

With a multiple trauma patient, *don't* use the head-tilt/chin-lift or head-tilt/neck-lift maneuvers to open his airway—you *must* suspect cervical spine injury until X-ray rules it out. Make sure your patient's secured to a backboard, and remember to immobilize his chest *first*. (If you immobilize his head first, you create a giant lever if his body moves before you stabilize it, possibly causing further serious injury.) Immobilize his head and neck by taping his forehead to the backboard or by applying a hard collar and sandbags.

Cardiac Emergency Assessment

If your patient's in a state of cardiac emergency, you'll want to assess his condition quickly and accurately. If your patient's *unconscious,* check his respiration and pulse. If necessary, institute cardiopulmonary resuscitation. Assess the *conscious* cardiac emergency patient as follows:

ASSESS CENTRAL PULSE

• Assess the patient's central pulse by palpating his carotid or femoral arteries. Check his pulse for regularity and rate. *Note:* A weak, rapid pulse may precede cardiac arrest.

• Assess for chest pain. If present, note its location, duration, and severity.

ASSESS CARDIAC RHYTHM

• Assess his cardiac rhythm by instituting cardiac monitoring. Suspect impaired perfusion if the patient has tachydysrhythmias or bradydysrhythmias.
  Before treating a dysrhythmia, remember to look at the patient; treat him, not the dysrhythmia. Also, when documenting the patient's cardiac rhythm, be sure to paste his rhythm strip on his chart.

ASSESS PERFUSION STATUS

• Assess his perfusion status by comparing central and peripheral pulses. Suspect impaired perfusion if the patient's peripheral pulse is weaker and/or slower than his central pulse.

• Measure his blood pressure. Remember, don't rule out shock just because hypotension's not evident.

• Determine his level of consciousness, and suspect shock if it's reduced.

• Check his skin; if it's cool and clammy, suspect impaired perfusion.

• Measure his urinary output. Consider shock confirmed if, along with the above findings, your patient's urinary output is severely decreased or absent.

Guide to Cardiac Emergencies

Do you know what emergency care to give in the following cardiac emergencies? The chart below will give you specific instructions. Study them carefully. In addition, remember these guidelines that apply to every cardiac emergency:

Call the doctor immediately. Make sure the patient has an open airway. Monitor him closely for signs of shock, and begin I.V. therapy, as needed, with the appropriate solution. Draw blood for type and cross matching in case your patient needs a blood transfusion. Get a complete medical history from the patient or his family, including information about the accident or injury (when applicable).

CARDIAC CONTUSION

Signs and symptoms:
• History of injury to anterior chest
• Ecchymosis on chest wall
• Retrosternal angina unrelieved by nitroglycerin but sometimes relieved by O_2 therapy
• Tachycardia
• EKG reading indicating *apparent* myocardial infarction or conduction disturbances
• Pericardial friction rub
• *Important:* In some cases, a patient with a cardiac contusion may be completely asymptomatic.

Special emergency nursing considerations:
• Follow the general guidelines listed in the introduction.
• Stay alert for signs of a ruptured aorta or ventricle, which may develop from this condition. Also watch for signs of cardiac tamponade. (You'll find complete details later in this chart.)
• Prepare patient for admission to the hospital. The doctor will want

him to have continuous EKG monitoring.

PENETRATING WOUND IN HEART

Signs and symptoms:
• In most cases, patient has a visible chest wound caused by an object like a knife or a bullet. However, heart penetration can occur from a bullet entering the abdomen or back.
• Chest pain, bleeding
• Drowsiness, loss of consciousness, possible agitation, combativeness, or confusion. (Note: Patient may appear intoxicated.)
• Tachycardia, muffled heart sounds, hypotension, dyspnea, increased central venous pressure (CVP), possible cardiac arrest
• Distended neck veins, although these may not be present immediately. For example, if the patient's in hypovolemic shock from blood loss, he may not have neck vein distention until he receives adequate I.V. fluid replacement.

Continued

Guide to Cardiac Emergencies
Continued

PENETRATING WOUND IN HEART

• Pneumothorax or hemothorax (may not develop until several hours after the injury).
Special emergency nursing considerations:
• Follow the general guidelines listed in the introduction.
• If a penetrating object is still in place when the patient arrives in the ED, don't remove it. Let it act as a seal for the damaged blood vessels and heart.
• Put patient on cardiac monitor.
• If the penetrating object's already been removed, control bleeding with direct pressure to the wound via a sterile cloth.
• Administer oxygen. Be prepared to intubate the patient if necessary.
• If the doctor decides to insert a chest tube, be ready to assist.
• Prepare patient for a thoracotomy.

CARDIAC TAMPONADE

(Fluid, blood, or blood clots trapped between the heart muscle and the pericardial sac or anterior chest wall)
Signs and symptoms:
• History of cardiac contusion, blunt trauma to anterior chest, penetrating chest wound, or recent cardiac surgery. *Important:*

Cardiac tamponade may also be a complication of an existing medical problem; for example, infectious pericardial neoplasm or uremia. In addition, tamponade may follow these procedures: cardiac catheterization or pacemaker insertion (from perforation of right heart ventricle), CPR, or diagnostic pericardial tap.
• Dyspnea
• Anxiety
• Pallor or cyanosis
• Agitation and neck vein distention
• Diaphoresis
• Weak, rapid, thready pulse or paradoxical pulse in which blood pressure drops on inspiration
• Muffled heart sounds
• Absent third heart sound
• Hypotension with narrowed pulse pressure
• Increased CVP
• Decreased urinary output
• Body position characteristic of cardiac tamponade, with the patient sitting upright and leaning forward
Special emergency nursing considerations:
• Your immediate concern is to maintain the patient's cardiac output until the intrapericardial pressure can be relieved. Follow the general guidelines listed in the introduction on the preceding page.

Continued

Guide to Cardiac Emergencies
Continued

CARDIAC TAMPONADE
Continued

• Prepare to assist the doctor with pericardiocentesis. Assemble the following equipment: pericardiocentesis tray, crash cart, I.V. fluids, endotracheal tubes, hand-held resuscitator, defibrillator, and cardiac pacemaker.
• Place patient on cardiac monitor.
• Check blood pressure, pulse, and respirations every 5 to 10 minutes. Don't rely totally on the cardiac monitor. The monitor may show normal heart rhythm and electrical conduction even when the heart's contractions and output are being impaired by increasing pressure in the pericardial sac (electromechanical dissociation).
• Administer oxygen.
• Following pericardiocentesis, prepare patient for a thoracotomy. As you do, observe him closely for recurring signs of tamponade, which may result in cardiac arrest.
• Watch for signs of pulmonary emboli: extreme agitation, dyspnea, pallor, combativeness, and chest pain. Notify the doctor immediately if they occur.

RUPTURED AORTA

Signs and symptoms:
• History of abrupt deceleration or compression injury
• Chest or back pain
• Dyspnea; weak, thready pulse; weakness in extremities; drowsiness, loss of consciousness
• In some cases, increased blood pressure and pulse amplitude in upper extremities, coupled with decreased blood pressure and pulse amplitude in lower extremities

Special emergency nursing considerations:
• Follow the general guidelines listed in the introduction on page 24.
• Prepare patient for immediate surgery.
• Administer oxygen and place patient on cardiac monitor.
• Have the following equipment nearby: tubes, hand-held resuscitator, and mechanical ventilator.
• Get ready to administer nitroprusside (Nipride*), according to doctor's order. Remember to protect the container from light.
• When you monitor patient's vital signs, pay particular attention to the pulses in his legs.

What Happens in Myocardial Infarction

Understanding the causes and pathophysiology of myocardial infarction (MI) will help you care for your patient more confidently. As you probably know, MI occurs when a portion of the cardiac muscle (myocardium) is deprived of oxygenated coronary blood flow, resulting in cellular ischemia, tissue injury, and then necrosis; irreversible myocardial damage ensues. Causes include:

• a buildup of atherosclerotic plaque (the major cause)
• coronary artery emboli
• coronary thrombosis
• hypertension
• massive hemorrhage
• coronary artery spasm.

When coronary artery blood flow is diminished, the heart pumps harder, increasing heart rate and blood pressure to meet increasing myocardial oxygen demands. Pulmonary circulation may back up in response to increased cardiac output, increasing the pressure needed to fill the atria. Dyspnea and fatigue result, further diminishing the heart's oxygen supply. The infarcted area alters the heart's contractile properties; this interferes with the ventricular relaxation period and the normal conduction system, creating irritable foci in the myocardium with a resulting decrease in cardiac output. The result may be heart failure, dysrhythmias, or cardiogenic shock.

Myocardial Damage Zones

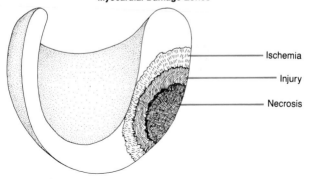

— Ischemia

— Injury

— Necrosis

How Various Kinds of Chest Pain Differ

	ONSET AND DURATION	LOCATION AND RADIATION
Myocardial infarction	Sudden onset; pain ½ to 2 hr; residual soreness, 1 to 3 days	Substernal, midline, or anterior chest pain; radiation down one or both arms to jaw, neck, or back
Angina (stable, unstable)	*Stable:* gradual onset; predictable pattern less than 30 min. *Unstable:* gradual onset; may occur or recur spontaneously; not relieved by nitroglycerin or rest	Substernal or anterior chest pain, not sharply localized; radiation to back, neck, arms, jaw, even upper abdomen or fingers
Pericarditis	Sudden onset; continuous pain lasting for days; residual soreness	Substernal pain to left of midline; radiation to back or subclavicular area
Pleuro-pulmonary	Gradual or sudden onset; continuous pain for hours	Pain over lung fields to side and back; radiation to anterior chest, shoulder, or neck
Esophageal-gastric	Gradual or sudden onset; continuous or intermittent	Substernal, midline, or anterior chest pain; radiation to upper abdomen, back, or shoulder
Musculo-skeletal	Gradual or sudden onset; continuous or intermittent	To right or left of midline

QUALITY AND INTENSITY	SIGNS AND SYMPTOMS	PRECIPITATING FACTORS
Severe pressure, deep sensation: "crushing," "stabbing," "viselike"	Apprehension, nausea, dyspnea, diaphoresis, increased pulse, decreased blood pressure, gallop heart sound	Occurrence at rest or with exertion (physical or emotional)
Mild-to-moderate pressure, uniform pattern of attacks; deep sensation, tightness, squeezing: "viselike"	Dyspnea, diaphoresis, nausea, desire to void, belching, apprehension; elevated blood pressure and increased heart rate immediately before or occuring at onset	Exertion, including sexual intercourse; stress; eating; micturition or defecation; cold or hot, humid weather
Mild ache to severe pain, deep or superficial: "stabbing," "knifelike"	Precordial friction rub; increased pain with movement, inspiration, left side position; decreased pain with leaning forward	Myocardial infarction or upper respiratory infection; no relation to effort
Deep sharp ache: "knifelike," "shooting," "crushing"	Pleural rub, fever, dyspnea; increased pain with inspiration and movement; decreased pain with sitting	Pneumonia or other respiratory infection
Squeezing pain, heartburn	Dysphagia, belching, reflux esophagitis; decreased pain with sitting or standing	Ingestion of alcohol or spicy foods, history of gastrointestinal problems
Soreness	Increased pain with movement	History of previous neck and arm injury

Identifying Life-Threatening EKG Waveforms

As you monitor your patient on a cardiac monitor or 12-lead EKG, watch for any of the waveforms below. They indicate that your patient faces an immediate life-threatening situation. Notify the doctor; then prepare to perform the nursing interventions described, if properly trained.

ELECTROMECHANICAL DISSOCIATION (EMD)
(Electrical conduction but no pulse)

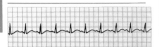

Characteristics:
• Organized electrical activity without any evidence of effective myocardial contraction
• Possible failure in the calcium transport system
• May mimic profound hypovolemia, cardiac tamponade, myocardial rupture, massive myocardial infarction, or tension pneumothorax

Interventions:
• Give CPR with optimal ventilation, as needed. Continue CPR if no palpable pulse is present. (Do this despite presence of rhythm.)
• Prepare to give epinephrine, sodium bicarbonate, and possibly calcium chloride, as ordered.
• Prepare to start an I.V. infusion of isoproterenol, as ordered, if EMD persists.

VENTRICULAR ASYSTOLE
(Cardiac standstill)

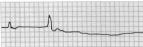

Characteristics:
• Totally absent ventricular electrical activity
• Possible P waves
• Possible severe metabolic deficit or extensive myocardial damage

Interventions:
• Begin CPR.
• Assist with endotracheal intubation.
• Start an I.V.
• Prepare to give epinephrine, sodium bicarbonate, atropine, calcium chloride, and isoproterenol, as ordered.
• Prepare to assist with temporary pacemaker insertion and defibrillation.

Continued

CARDIOPULMONARY EMERGENCIES

Identifying Life-Threatening EKG Waveforms
Continued

CARDIOPULMONARY EMERGENCIES

VENTRICULAR FIBRILLATION

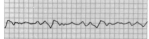

Characteristics:
• May arise spontaneously or be triggered by premature ventricular contractions or ventricular tachycardia
• Ventricular rhythm rapid and chaotic; QRS complexes not identifiable
• Patient unconscious at onset
• Absent pulses, heart sounds, and blood pressure
• Dilated pupils and cyanosis
• Possible convulsions
• Possible death of patient within minutes (ventricular fibrillation is the most common cause of sudden death in patients with coronary heart disease)

Interventions:
• Give precordial thump, if patient is monitored.
• Defibrillate the patient.
• Begin CPR.
• Administer epinephrine and sodium bicarbonate, as ordered.
• Prepare to give lidocaine or bretylium to treat myocardial irritability and to prevent recurring dysrhythmias.

VENTRICULAR TACHYCARDIA

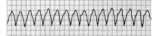

Characteristics:
• Three or more ventricular beats occurring in succession, with a ventricular rate greater than 100
• Decreased cardiac output

Interventions:
• Perform precordial thump if patient's pulseless and on a monitor.
• Prepare to give lidocaine.
• Prepare to cardiovert if lidocaine's ineffective and patient's unconscious.
• Administer lidocaine drip, procainamide, and bretylium, as ordered.
• Suspect electrolyte imbalance if the patient's tachycardia returns despite antiarrhythmic drug therapy.
• Suspect lactic acidosis if tachycardia persists for more than 5 minutes; prepare to give sodium bicarbonate.
• Prepare to assist with temporary pacemaker insertion for recurrent tachycardia.

Continued

Identifying Life-Threatening EKG Waveforms
Continued

CARDIOPULMONARY
EMERGENCIES

PREMATURE VENTRICULAR CONTRACTIONS (PVCs)

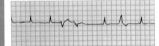

Characteristics:
● Longer-than-normal pause may occur immediately after premature beats (compensatory pause)
● Indicator of myocardial irritability or electrolyte imbalance
● May initiate ventricular tachycardia, then ventricular fibrillation when they occur *frequently* (six or more times/minute), strike on the T wave of preceding complex (R on T pattern), have more than one configuration (multifocal PVCs), occur sequentially for two or more beats
● Bigeminy: when every second beat is a PVC
● Trigeminy: pattern of two normal beats followed by a PVC

Interventions:
● Prepare to give lidocaine (sometimes procainamide or potassium) as ordered to suppress irritable ventricular focus.

● Diuretic therapy can cause PVCs; anticipate giving potassium to restore electrolyte balance and to correct drug-induced ectopic beats.
● Watch the patient for signs and symptoms of lidocaine overdose, such as seizures.
● With procainamide, monitor the patient for hypotension.

SYMPTOMATIC SUPRAVEN-TRICULAR TACHYCARDIA (SVT)

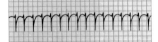

Characteristics:
● Unusually rapid rhythms arising in sinus, atrial, or atrioventricular junctional tissue
● Decreases cardiac output due to rapid ventricular response rate, ineffective atrial contraction, or abnormal contraction sequence

Continued

Identifying Life-Threatening EKG Waveforms
Continued

SYMPTOMATIC SUPRAVENTRICULAR TACHYCARDIA (SVT)
Continued

• Reentrant atrial tachycardia, ectopic atrial tachycardia, multifocal atrial tachycardia, atrial fibrillation and atrial flutter with rapid ventricular response, paroxysmal atrial tachycardia, and nonparoxysmal junctional tachycardia may be interpreted as SVT

Interventions:
• Prepare to give I.V. verapamil, Inderal, and digoxin as ordered.
• Prepare to cardiovert.

SYMPTOMATIC BRADYCARDIA

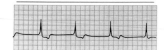

Characteristics:
• Bradydysrhythmias, possibly including sinus bradycardia, junctional rhythm, idioventricular rhythm, heart block
• Possible ectopic rhythms
• Reduced threshold for ventricular fibrillation, possible decreased cardiac output

Interventions:
• Start an I.V. and prepare to give atropine, then isoproterenol, as ordered.

• Assist with temporary pacemaker insertion, as ordered, if the patient's heartbeat doesn't respond to drugs.
• Restore volume status if dysrhythmia was caused by hypotension.

COMPLETE HEART BLOCK
(Third-degree AV block)

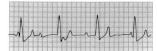

Characteristics:
• Slow, regular, steady heartbeat
• Possible episodes of syncope and convulsions, left ventricular failure
• Cardiac output insufficient to meet circulatory demands
• Potential cessation of ventricular impulse or replacement by irritable ventricular foci

Interventions:
• Prepare to assist with temporary pacemaker insertion.
• Prepare to give atropine, as ordered.
• Prepare to give an infusion of isoproterenol, as ordered.
• Be prepared to defibrillate, if necessary.

Heart Failure: Signs and Symptoms

LEFT HEART FAILURE

- Elevated blood pressure
- Paroxysmal nocturnal dyspnea, dyspnea on exertion, orthopnea
- Bronchial wheezing
- Hypoxia, respiratory acidosis
- Rales
- Cough with frothy pink sputum
- Cyanosis or pallor
- Third or fourth heart sounds
- Palpitations, dysrhythmias, tachycardia
- Elevated pulmonary artery diastolic and pulmonary capillary wedge pressures
- Pulsus alternans
- Oliguria

RIGHT HEART FAILURE

- Weakness, fatigue, dizziness, syncope
- Hepatomegaly, with or without pain
- Ascites
- Dependent pitting peripheral edema
- Jugular vein distention
- Hepatojugular reflux
- Oliguria
- Dysrhythmias, tachycardia
- Elevated central venous/right atrial pressure
- Nausea, vomiting, anorexia, abdominal distention
- Weight gain
- Splenomegaly (uncommon)

What Happens in Congestive Heart Failure

Congestive heart failure (CHF) occurs when cardiac output is inadequate to meet the body's needs. The resulting inadequate cardiac output, venous pressure increase, and arterial pressure decrease trigger a series of compensatory mechanisms designed to ensure perfusion of vital organs.

When compensation efforts fail, heart failure typically occurs in the left ventricle first (causing pulmonary congestion) and then progresses to the right ventricle (causing visceral and tissue congestion).

Managing Pulmonary Edema

INITIAL STAGE

Symptoms:
- Persistent cough
- Slight dyspnea/orthopnea
- Exercise intolerance
- Restlessness and anxiety
- Crepitant rales at lung bases
- Diastolic gallop

Nursing responsibilities:
- Check color and amount of expectoration.
- Position patient for comfort.
- Auscultate chest for rales and S_3.
- Medicate, as ordered.
- Monitor apical and radial pulses.
- Assist patient with all needs, to conserve strength.
- Provide emotional support (through all stages) for patient and family.

ACUTE STAGE

Symptoms:
- Acute shortness of breath
- Respirations—rapid, noisy (audible wheeze, rales)
- Cough—more intense and productive of frothy, blood-tinged sputum
- Cyanosis—cold, clammy skin
- Tachycardia—dysrhythmias
- Hypotension

Nursing responsibilities:
- Give oxygen (preferably by high-concentration mask or IPPB).
- Insert I.V., if not already done.
- Aspirate nasopharynx, as needed.
- Apply rotating tourniquets.
- Give digitalis, morphine, and potent diuretics (e.g., furosemide), as ordered.
- Insert Foley catheter.
- Calculate intake and output accurately.
- Draw blood to measure arterial blood gases.
- Attach cardiac monitor leads and observe EKG.
- Prepare for phlebotomy, if necessary.
- Keep resuscitation equipment available.

ADVANCED STAGE

Symptoms:
- Decreased level of consciousness
- Ventricular dysrhythmias; shock
- Diminished breath sounds

Nursing responsibilities:
- Be prepared for cardioversion.
- Assist with intubation and mechanical ventilation, and resuscitate if necessary.

Understanding Cardiac Emergency Drugs

During a code, seconds are crucial and the margin for error is narrow. You can increase your effectiveness during a code by making sure you're familiar with the drugs used to treat life-threatening cardiac conditions. You need to know each drug's mechanism of action, usual dose, and route of administration. The chart below provides this information, along with important nursing considerations.

ATROPINE SULFATE

Indications:
• Excessive vagus-induced brady-cardia, first degree atrioventricular (AV) block, and Mobitz I AV block

Mechanism of action:
Cholinergic blocker (parasympa-tholytic)

Dose/route:
• I.V. push: administer 0.5 to 1 mg over 1 to 2 minutes. Can be repeated every 5 minutes; total dose should not exceed 2 mg.

Nursing considerations:
• Lower doses (less than 0.5 mg) may cause bradycardia.
• Higher doses (more than 2 mg) may cause full vagal blockage.
• Contraindicated for glaucoma patients (isoproterenol should be used instead).
• May increase ischemic area in patients with acute myocardial in-farction (MI); use only if bradycar-dia is severe and symptomatic.
• Monitor cardiac rhythm for heart rate greater than 110 beats/min-ute and for premature ventricular contractions (PVCs).
• Monitor for urine retention.
• Maintain hydration and oral moisture.

BRETYLIUM TOSYLATE (BRETYLOL, BRETYLATE**)

Indications:
• Ventricular dysrhythmias that are unresponsive to lidocaine

Mechanism of action:
Antiarrhythmic

Dose/route:
• I.V. push: rapidly administer 5 mg/kg; can be repeated every 15 to 30 minutes until 30 mg/kg has been given.
• Infusion: 500 mg diluted to at least 50 ml with dextrose 5% in water (D_5W) or normal saline so-lution; infuse at 1 to 2 mg/minute

Nursing considerations:
• Generally not used to treat PVCs unless other drugs fail.
• May increase digitalis toxicity.
• May potentiate hypotension.
• Keep your patient supine to minimize orthostatic changes.
• Be prepared for vomiting after rapid administration of undiluted drug.
• Monitor blood pressure, pulse, and cardiac rhythm.

**Available in Canada only.

Continued

Understanding Cardiac Emergency Drugs
Continued

CARDIOPULMONARY
EMERGENCIES

CALCIUM CHLORIDE

Indications:
- Asystole and electromechanical dissociation of the heart
- Hyperkalemia

Mechanism of action:
Electrolyte

Dose/route:
- I.V. push: administer 5 to 10 ml at 1 ml/minute; can be repeated every 10 minutes.
- Infusion: can add to D_5W or normal saline solution; flow rate should not exceed 1.5 mEq/minute.

Nursing considerations:
- Contraindicated in patients with hypercalcemia.
- Infiltration may produce severe tissue damage.
- Use cautiously in patients receiving digoxin; may cause dysrhythmias.
- Do not give to patients with high serum phosphate levels; may produce fatal calcium phosphate deposits in vital organs.
- Do not mix with any other medications—it will precipitate.
- Monitor patient for normal serum calcium levels (8.5 to 10.5 mg/100 ml, or 4.5 to 5.8 mEq/liter)
- Remind the doctor if your patient is receiving digoxin.
- Monitor for bradycardia and for decreased QT interval.

DIGOXIN (LANOXIN*, MASOXIN)

Indications:
- Atrial fibrillation and flutter, paroxysmal atrial tachycardia, and congestive heart failure (CHF)

Mechanism of action:
Cardiotonic glycoside

Dose/route:
- I.V. push: administer 0.5 to 1 mg divided over 24 hours, then 0.125 to 0.5 mg daily.

Nursing considerations:
- Toxic levels may cause life-threatening dysrhythmias, hypotension, or severe CHF.
- Do not administer calcium salts to a digitalized patient.
- Use with caution in elderly patients and patients with MI, incomplete AV block, renal insufficiency, or hypothyroidism.
- Do not administer to patients with ventricular tachycardia (unless caused by CHF or ventricular fibrillation).
- Monitor EKG, blood pressure, electrolytes, blood urea nitrogen, and serum creatinine.
- Monitor the serum digoxin level.
- Obtain a 12-lead EKG to document significant changes in cardiac rate or rhythm.
- Withhold 1 to 2 days before performing cardioversion.

*Available in U.S. and Canada.

Continued

Understanding Cardiac Emergency Drugs
Continued

DOBUTAMINE HYDROCHLORIDE (DOBUTREX)

Indications:
• Used in short-term treatment to increase cardiac output in cardiogenic shock and heart failure
Mechanism of action:
Adrenergic (sympathomimetic)
Dose/route:
• Infusion: reconstitute with D_5W or normal saline solution, then prepare standard dilution; administer 2.5 to 10 mcg/kg/minute.
Nursing considerations:
• Don't use with beta blockers, such as propranolol.
• Incompatible with alkaline solutions.
• Patients with atrial fibrillation should receive digoxin first, to prevent rapid ventricular response.
• Infiltration may produce severe tissue damage.
• Monitor blood pressure, central venous pressure (CVP), pulmonary capillary wedge pressure (PCWP), cardiac rhythm, and urine output.
• Always use an infusion pump.

DOPAMINE HYDROCHLORIDE (INTROPIN*)

Indications:
• Cardiogenic shock and other hemodynamic problems, hypotension, and decreased cardiac output
Mechanism of action:
Adrenergic (sympathomimetic)
Dose/route:
• Infusion: standard dilution; may use with D_5W, dextrose 5% in normal saline solution, or dextrose 5% in ½ normal saline solution; administer 2 to 5 mcg/kg/minute, up to 50 mcg/kg/minute.
Nursing considerations:
• May precipitate dysrhythmias.
• Infiltration may produce severe tissue damage.
• Solution deteriorates after 24 hours.
• Don't mix other drugs in bottle.
• Don't give alkaline drugs through the same I.V. line as dopamine.
• Titrate to maintain desired systolic blood pressure and urine output.
• Always use an infusion pump.
• Monitor patient's cardiac rhythm, urine output, blood pressure, CVP, and PCWP.
• Use a large vein to minimize risk of severe tissue damage from extravasation.

*Available in U.S. and Canada.

Continued

Understanding Cardiac Emergency Drugs
Continued

EPINEPHRINE HYDROCHLO-RIDE (ADRENALIN CHLORIDE)

Indications:
• Asystole and ventricular fibrillation
Mechanism of action:
Adrenergic (sympathomimetic)
Dose/route:
• I.V. push: administer 5 to 10 ml of 1:10,000 solution (0.5 to 1 mg) over 1 minute.
• Intracardiac: administer 1 to 10 ml of 1:10,000 solution (0.1 to 1 mg).
• Intratracheal: instill 1 to 2 mg per 10 ml sterile water (1 ml of 1:10,000, or 1 ml of 1:5,000) directly into endotracheal tube.
• Infusion: can mix 2 to 4 mg in 500 ml D_5W; administer at 1 to 4 mcg/minute.
Nursing considerations:
• Increases intraocular pressure.
• May exacerbate CHF, dysrhythmias, angina pectoris, hyperthyroidism, and emphysema.
• May cause headache, tremors, or palpitations.
• Monitor blood pressure every 2 to 5 minutes until it's stable.
• Monitor cardiac rhythm.
• Watch for signs of overdose: cold and diaphoretic skin, cyanosis of nail beds, tachypnea, and changes in mental status. If any occur, discontinue the drug immediately.

ISOPROTERENOL HYDRO-CHLORIDE (ISOPRENALINE, ISUPREL*)**

Indications:
• Complete heart block, asystole, and cardiogenic shock
Mechanism of action:
Adrenergic (sympathomimetic)
Dose/route:
• Infusion: use standard dilution; administer at 0.5 to 20 mcg/minute and titrate as needed.
Nursing considerations:
• Use cautiously in patients with heart failure.
• Don't administer with epinephrine.
• Use cautiously when administering together with propranolol.
• Don't administer for preexisting dysrhythmias induced by digitalis toxicity.
• Monitor intraarterial pressure, if possible.
• Using an infusion pump, titrate as ordered.
• Check blood pressure every 2 to 3 minutes until stable.
• Monitor CVP and PCWP.
• Record urine output hourly.

*Available in U.S. and Canada.
**Available in Canada only.

Continued

CARDIOPULMONARY EMERGENCIES

Understanding Cardiac Emergency Drugs
Continued

LIDOCAINE HYDROCHLORIDE
(LIGNOCAINE**, XYLOCAINE*)

Indications:
• PVCs and ventricular tachycardia
Mechanism of action:
Antiarrhythmic
Dose/route:
• I.V. push: administer 50 to 100 mg; can be repeated every 5 minutes; total dose should not exceed 200 mg.
• Infusion: standard dilution; administer at 1 to 4 mg/minute.
• Intratracheal: infuse 50 to 100 mg per 10 ml sterile water.
Nursing considerations:
• Don't mix with sodium bicarbonate.
• Don't use if your patient has a high-grade sinoatrial or AV block.
• Discontinue if PR interval or QRS complex widens, or if dysrhythmias worsen.
• Use cautiously in patients with severe renal or liver impairment.
• May lead to ventricular tachycardia if used to correct PVCs resulting from bradycardia.
• May lead to central nervous system (CNS) toxicity, especially in patients with heart failure.
• Titrate as ordered to control dysrhythmias.

*Available in U.S. and Canada.
**Available in Canada only.

• Observe patient frequently for signs of CNS toxicity: numbness of lips, face, or tongue; tremors; paresthesia; blurred or double vision; dizziness; tinnitus; and seizures. If any occur, stop the infusion and treat the toxicity.
• Monitor cardiac rhythm constantly.
• Monitor blood pressure every 10 to 15 minutes until stable; slow infusion if hypotension occurs.

NOREPINEPHRINE INJECTION
(formerly levarterenol bitartrate)
(LEVOPHED*)

Indications:
• Acute hypotensive states
Mechanism of action:
Adrenergic (sympathomimetic)
Dose/route:
Infusion: initially, 8 to 12 mcg/minute I.V., then adjust to maintain normal blood pressure. Average maintenance dose 2 to 4 mcg/minute.
Nursing considerations:
• Not a substitute for blood or fluid volume deficit. If deficit exists, it should be replaced before vasopressors are administered.

Continued

Understanding Cardiac Emergency Drugs
Continued

• Norepinephrine solutions deteriorate after 24 hours. Discard after that time.
• Use large vein, as in antecubital fossa, to minimize risk of extravasation. Check site frequently for signs of extravasation. If it occurs, stop infusion immediately and call doctor. He may counteract effect by infiltrating area with 5 to 10 mg phentolamine and 10 to 15 ml normal saline solution.
• Keep emergency drugs on hand to reverse effects of norepinephrine: atropine for reflex bradycardia; propranolol for dysrhythmias; phentolamine for increased vasopressor effects.
• Administer in dextrose and saline solution; saline solution alone is not recommended.

PROCAINAMIDE HYDROCHLORIDE (PRONESTYL*)

Indications:
• PVCs and ventricular fibrillation when lidocaine isn't effective
Mechanism of action:
Antiarrhythmic
Dose/route:
• I.V. push: administer 100 mg at 20 mg/minute; can be repeated every 5 minutes; total dose shouldn't exceed 1 g.
• Infusion: infuse 2 to 6 mg/minute.

*Available in U.S. and Canada.

Nursing considerations:
• Can cause precipitous hypotension; don't use for treating second- or third-degree heart block unless a pacemaker's been inserted.
• Can cause AV block and PVCs that may result in ventricular fibrillation.
• Monitor blood pressure continuously.
• Monitor EKG for widening QRS complexes.
• Maintain a slow administration rate to avoid serious hypotension.
• Always use an infusion pump.

PROPRANOLOL HYDROCHLORIDE (INDERAL*)

Indications:
• Supraventricular, ventricular, and atrial dysrhythmias and excessive tachydysrhythmias
Mechanism of action:
Beta blocker
Dose/route:
• I.V. push: administer 1 to 3 mg at a rate not greater than 1 mg/minute; may be repeated in 2 minutes.
Nursing considerations:
• Can alter requirements for insulin and oral hypoglycemic drugs.
• Can cause excessive bradycardia.

Continued

CARDIOPULMONARY EMERGENCIES

Understanding Cardiac Emergency Drugs
Continued

• Use cautiously when administering with isoproterenol and aminophylline (exaggerates beta-blocking effect).
• Monitor EKG, heart rate, and rhythm frequently.
• Monitor for hypoglycemia.
• Auscultate for rales, gallop rhythm, and third or fourth heart sounds.

SODIUM BICARBONATE

Indications:
• Cardiac arrest
Mechanism of action:
Alkalizer
Dose/route:
• I.V. push: rapidly administer 44.6 mEq in 50 ml D_5W (1 mEq/kg); repeat doses according to arterial blood gas values.
Nursing considerations:
• Don't mix with epinephrine; causes epinephrine degradation.
• Don't mix with calcium salts; forms insoluble precipitates.
• After injection, thoroughly flush the line with I.V. fluid.
• Monitor arterial pH.

VERAPAMIL (ISOPTIN*, CALAN)

Indications:
• Supraventricular tachydysrhythmias
Mechanism of action:
Calcium channel blocker
Dose/route:
• I.V. push: administer 5 to 10 mg (0.075 to 0.15 mg/kg) over a minimum of 2 minutes; for older patients, administer over 3 minutes; can be repeated in 30 minutes.
Nursing considerations:
• Contraindicated in patients with hypotension, cardiogenic shock, severe CHF, and second- or third-degree AV block.
• High doses or overly rapid administration can cause a significant drop in blood pressure.
• Monitor cardiac rhythm for AV block and bradycardia.
• Monitor blood pressure.

*Available in U.S. and Canada.

Highlighting Streptokinase

If streptokinase is administered to a patient with an acute myocardial infarction, his chances of survival and recovery may improve. Here's why:

Streptokinase is a thrombolytic, so it dissolves the clot occluding the artery. This improves myocardial perfusion and, if the drug's given within 3 to 4 hours of the onset of the patient's chest pain, it limits the infarction's size.

Administering streptokinase directly into the occluded coronary artery, using angiography in a cardiac catheterization laboratory, is the most effective treatment. (You may also give streptokinase by continuous I.V. for such disorders as pulmonary emboli and deep-vein thrombosis.)

Remember these important points about administering streptokinase:

• Always establish a perfusion baseline of peripheral pulses.
• Before infusion, double-check all doses and infusion rates with another nurse.
• Don't give intramuscular or intravenous injections during infusion or for 24 hours afterward.
• Establish two I.V. lines before infusion. Use one for streptokinase, the second for any other drugs you need to give.
• Inspect the infusion site hourly for signs of bleeding. After infusion, inspect the site every 15 minutes the first hour, every 30 minutes for 2 to 8 hours, then once per shift.
• Monitor and document the following every hour, before and after infusion: the patient's pulses and color, and the sensitivity of his affected and unaffected limbs.
• Keep a laboratory flow sheet so you can monitor the following during and after infusion: partial thromboplastin time, prothrombin time, hemoglobin, and hematocrit.
• Monitor carefully, for dysrhythmias, any patient receiving intracoronary streptokinase for lysis of coronary artery thrombi.
• Test all the patient's nasogastric aspirate and his stools and urine for blood, during and after infusion.
• Apply direct pressure to the infusion site for at least 30 minutes after the catheter's removed.
• Watch the patient for flushing, itching, urticaria, headaches and muscle aches, and nausea. These may indicate a mild allergic and febrile reaction.

Recognizing Digitalis Toxicity

Digitalis' therapeutic range is narrow—in some patients even a therapeutic dose may be toxic. Of course, this is why toxicity from digitalis glycosides is relatively common in patients taking the drug.

Patients taking digitalis preparations who are also taking certain other drugs, or who have certain disorders, are at particularly high risk for developing toxicity.

Examples include:

• the patient with reduced renal function who's taking digoxin
• the patient with reduced hepatic function who's taking digitoxin
• the patient with electrolyte imbalances, myocardial infarction, pulmonary disease, or hypothyroidism
• the patient on quinidine or verapamil therapy.

If you suspect your patient's developing toxicity, discontinue digitalis and notify the doctor. He may order antiarrhythmic drugs and a temporary pacemaker. Also, he may discontinue diuretics, which contribute to potassium loss (hypokalemia), and take action to correct electrolyte imbalances.

Expect the doctor to discontinue the digitalis or to readjust the dosage. If you suspect an intentional overdose, assess the patient's mental status—his disease may be causing suicidal depression.

Watch your patient for signs and symptoms of digitalis toxicity, listed below.

Note: Digitalis toxicity affects the cardiovascular system and other body systems. So nausea, vomiting, and anorexia commonly accompany toxicity—especially in geriatric patients. But digitalis-induced dysrhythmias may occur *without* any other signs and symptoms.

SIGNS AND SYMPTOMS

Most common:

• Anorexia
• Nausea, vomiting
• Malaise
• Headache
• Ventricular ectopic beats
• Premature ventricular contractions (bigeminy)
• Bradycardia

Less common:

• Blurred vision
• Headache
• Yellow cast to vision or halos seen around lights
• Disorientation
• Diarrhea
• Ventricular tachycardia
• Sinoatrial and atrioventricular block
• Ventricular fibrillation

Hypertensive Crisis

Hypertensive crisis is an acute, life-threatening rise in blood pressure (diastolic usually over 120 mm Hg). It may develop in hypertensive patients after abrupt discontinuation of antihypertensive medication; increased salt consumption; increased production of renin, epinephrine, and norepinephrine; and added stress. This emergency requires immediate and vigorous treatment to lower blood pressure and thereby prevent cerebrovascular accident, left heart failure, and pulmonary edema.

Hypertensive crisis produces severe and widespread symptoms, including headache, drowsiness, mental clouding, vomiting, focal neurologic signs (such as paresthesias), and, if pulmonary edema is present, shortness of breath and hemoptysis. Treatment to rapidly lower blood pressure and thereby prevent hypertensive encephalopathy may include vasodilators, such as I.V. nitroprusside, hydralazine, or diazoxide; a potent diuretic, such as furosemide; and a sympathetic blocker, such as methyldopa, trimethaphan, or phentolamine.

In the early stages of antihypertensive I.V. therapy, monitor blood pressure and heart rate frequently (as often as every 1 to 3 minutes with some drugs) for a precipitous drop, indicating hypersensitivity to the prescribed medications. Maintain blood pressure level, as ordered.

Keep the patient calm; if he's excited, administer a sedative, as ordered. Record intake and output accurately, and, if necessary, explain the reasons for fluid restriction. Watch closely for hypotension, and, until blood pressure is stable at a desirable level, check for signs of heart failure, such as tachycardia, tachypnea, dyspnea, pulmonary rales, S_3 or S_4 gallops, neck vein distention, cyanosis, and edema.

Initial Respiratory Assessment Checklist
Assess the ABCs first and intervene appropriately.

CHECK FOR:

• stridor or inability to talk, indicating airway obstruction
• cyanosis, indicating tissue hypoxia
• changes in mental status (apprehension, anxiety, agitation, confusion, restlessness, lethargy, or unconsciousness may indicate hypoxemia)
• severe chest pain and guarded posture, which restrict breathing and may indicate injury.

INTERVENE BY:

• administering oxygen (respiratory emergencies cause poor gas exchange).

PREPARE FOR:

• chest tube insertion
• assisted ventilation
• endotracheal intubation.

Special Consideration

Pediatric patients with respiratory emergencies require your special attention. Be particularly alert to upper airway obstruction in infants and young children, who commonly aspirate small foreign objects, such as buttons and parts of toys. Remember, too, that a very young child's tongue occupies a proportionately larger space in his mouth and pharynx than in an adult's. So, to clear his airway when his tongue's blocking it, you'll need to use the jaw thrust maneuver or an oral airway. If you're assisting with endotracheal tube insertion, *don't* severely hyperextend the child's neck. Why? Because you may occlude his airway completely. Gentle extension (the "sniff" position) is all a pediatric patient requires.

   With a young child, stridor occurring with fever and drooling may indicate *epiglottitis*—a life-threatening condition that can totally obstruct the airway. If you or the doctor suspect epiglottitis, *don't* inspect the pharynx directly: this can cause laryngospasm, increasing edema, and asphyxiation.

Assessing Breath Sounds

As part of your emergency assessment, percuss and auscultate your patient's chest. *Percussion* helps you identify compressed lung tissue or fluid or tissue that's replaced air in the alveoli. *Auscultation* helps you determine whether your patient has a bronchial obstruction or air or fluid in his lungs.

Normal breath sounds are described as bronchial (tubular), bronchovesicular, and vesicular. Crackles (rales), wheezes (sibilant rhonchi), rhonchi (sonorous rhonchi), stridor, and pleural friction rub are adventitious (abnormal) breath sounds. You may hear abnormal breath sounds superimposed over normal ones.

The chart below will help you identify abnormal breath sounds associated with respiratory disorders.

DISORDER	PERCUS-SION	CHANGES IN NORMAL BREATH SOUNDS	ADVENTI-TIOUS BREATH SOUNDS
Consolida-tion	Dull	High-pitched, bronchial	Fine crackles early; coarse crackles later
Atelectasis	Dull	Diminished or absent; high-pitched, bronchial	Fine crackles early; coarse crackles later
Pleural effu-sion or em-pyema	Dull to absent	Diminished or absent; high-pitched, bronchial	Pleural friction rub

Continued

Assessing Breath Sounds
Continued

DISORDER	PERCUS-SION	CHANGES IN NORMAL BREATH SOUNDS	ADVENTI-TIOUS BREATH SOUNDS
Pneumo-thorax	Normal or hyperreso-nant	Diminished or absent; high-pitched, bronchial	Fine crackles when fluid present
Acute or chronic bronchitis	Normal	Vesicular with pro-longed expi-ration	Rhonchi; coarse crackles
Bronchial asthma	Normal or hyperreso-nant	Vesicular with pro-longed expi-ration	Wheezes
Pulmonary edema	Normal or dull	Bronchial or vesicular	Coarse crackles

Special Consideration

Realize that breath sounds can be affected by inadvertent placement of an endotracheal tube into the right mainstem bronchus. This causes decreased breath sounds on the patient's left side. To check that a tube's placed correctly, auscultate the patient's chest to be sure his breath sounds are equal on both sides.

Allen's Test: Your First Priority

Your patient needs an arterial line or arterial blood gas measurements *now*. Despite the urgency, do the Allen's test first. Why? Because these procedures invade the radial artery and may damage it. Since the hand's only other main blood source is the ulnar artery, you need to make sure that's patent *before* the procedure. Here's how:

• Have your patient clench his fist. Next, compress his radial and ulnar arteries.

• Have him unclench his fist. His palm will blanch because you're stopping the blood flow.

• Release pressure from the ulnar artery *only*. If blood flow's adequate, his palm will flush within 5 seconds. If blood flow's inadequate, you'll have to find another insertion site.

How Respiratory Disorders Affect ABGs

Arterial blood gas (ABG) tests help you assess your patient's respiratory status and monitor his therapy.

ABG tests evaluate gas exchange in your patient's lungs by measuring the partial pressures of oxygen (PaO_2), carbon dioxide ($PaCO_2$), and pH in arterial blood samples. For example, a low PaO_2 level indicates he's hypoxemic and may need oxygen. Subsequent PaO_2 measurements monitor the effectiveness of his oxygen therapy.

A rise in $PaCO_2$ indicates he's hypoventilating and retaining carbon dioxide, whereas a drop in $PaCO_2$ indicates he's hyperventilating and losing too much carbon dioxide. In both situations, he may need mechanical ventilation. You can monitor the mechanical ventilation's effectiveness by noting the patient's $PaCO_2$ levels on serial ABGs.

Respiratory Acidosis

Alveolar hypoventilation causes respiratory retention of CO_2, leading to carbonic acid excess and a decreased pH. Arterial PCO_2 above 45 mm Hg and pH below 7.35 characterize respiratory acidosis.

PREDISPOSING FACTORS

- Airway obstruction
- Chest-wall injury
- Neuromuscular disease
- Drug overdose (CNS depression)
- ARDS
- Pneumothorax
- Pneumonia
- Pulmonary edema

SIGNS AND SYMPTOMS

- Tachycardia
- Shallow, slow respirations
- Dyspnea
- Dysrhythmias
- Cyanosis
- Diaphoresis
- Lethargy
- Confusion
- $PCO_2 > 45$;
  pH < 7.35; but
  HCO_3 22 to 26 (normal)

TREATMENT GOAL

Effective treatment tries to correct the underlying source of alveolar hypoventilation.

INTERVENTION

- Be alert for critical changes in the patient's respiratory, CNS, and cardiovascular functions. Report any such changes immediately.
- Give O_2 (use low concentrations in patients with chronic obstructive pulmonary disease).
- Give intravenous fluids.
- Give inhaled or intravenous bronchodilators.
- Start mechanical ventilation if hypoventilation can't be corrected immediately.
- Monitor ABGs and electrolytes.

Respiratory Alkalosis

Alveolar hyperventilation causes excess exhalation of CO_2, leading to carbonic acid deficit and an elevated pH. Arterial PCO_2 below 35 mm Hg and pH above 7.45 characterize respiratory alkalosis.

PREDISPOSING FACTORS

• Extreme anxiety
• CNS injury to respiratory center
• Fever
• Overventilation during mechanical ventilation
• Pulmonary embolism
• Congestive heart failure
• Salicylate intoxication (early)

SIGNS AND SYMPTOMS

• Tachycardia
• Deep, rapid breathing
• Light-headedness
• Numbness and tingling or arm and leg paresthesias
• Carpopedal spasm
• Tetany
• $PCO_2 < 35$; pH > 7.45; but HCO_3 22 to 26 (normal)

TREATMENT GOAL

Treatment tries to eradicate the underlying condition; for example, fever or sepsis.

INTERVENTIONS

• Observe the patient carefully for subtle changes in neurologic, neuromuscular, or cardiovascular functions. Report any such changes immediately.
• Have the patient breathe into a paper bag. (Rebreathing his CO_2 increases his PCO_2.)
• Administer sedatives and give calm, reassuring support. (Hyperventilation is often triggered by anxiety attacks.)
• Perform gastric lavage if salicylate overdose caused the alkalosis.
• Monitor ABGs and electrolytes.

Guide to Pulmonary Emergencies

Use the chart below for specific instructions to follow in a pulmonary emergency. Also keep in mind these general guidelines: Call the doctor immediately. Make sure the patient has an open airway. Monitor him closely for signs of shock, and begin I.V. therapy, as needed, with the appropriate solution. Draw blood for type and cross matching in case he needs a blood transfusion. Get a complete medical history from the patient or his family, including information about the accident or injury (when applicable).

PNEUMOTHORAX

Signs and symptoms:
• History of blunt chest trauma caused by fall, blow, violent cough, or sudden deceleration
• History of penetrating chest injury, such as a knife or bullet wound. May also be a complication caused by CVP line insertion or thoracentesis
• Possible sudden sharp chest pain, sometimes referred to shoulder, opposite side of chest, or abdomen
• Dyspnea, dry, hacking cough, diminished or absent breath sounds on affected side, asymmetric chest movements
• Hyperresonance on percussion
• Possible subcutaneous emphysema (crepitus) on neck or chest wall
Special emergency nursing considerations:
• Maintain an open airway.
• Monitor for signs of shock and begin I.V. therapy, as ordered.
• Draw blood for type and cross matching in case your patient needs a blood transfusion.

• Take a complete history from the patient or family, including information about the injury.
• If patient has a penetrating chest wound, prepare to assist the doctor with immediate insertion of flutter valve or chest tube.
• If the patient needs oxygen, administer it with a nasal cannula or face mask, at 4 to 10 liters per minute. If your patient has chronic obstructive pulmonary disease (COPD), administer oxygen at 2 liters (or less) per minute.
• Prepare to intubate the COPD patient, if necessary.
• Watch for signs of mediastinal shift.

HEMOTHORAX
(blood in pleural space)

Signs and symptoms:
• History of trauma to chest wall, lung tissue, or mediastinum; pleural or pulmonary neoplasm; pulmonary infarction; or pleural tear from spontaneous pneumothorax. May also be a complication of anticoagulant therapy after chest surgery.

Continued

Guide to Pulmonary Emergencies
Continued

HEMOTHORAX
Continued

• Chest pain; dyspnea; tachycardia; diaphoresis; hypotension; skin color changes; asymmetric chest movements (if hemothorax is large); frothy or bloody sputum; weak, thready pulse; rapid, shallow respirations; possible cyanosis; EKG changes; and ecchymosis over affected area
• Diminished or absent breath sounds on affected side; dullness on percussion
• Possible rib or sternum fracture
Special emergency nursing considerations:
• Follow the general guidelines listed on the page 52.
• Administer oxygen by nasal cannula or mask.
• Be ready to help doctor with chest tube insertion. After the chest tube's inserted, record the initial amount of bloody drainage on the patient's chart. If it exceeds 1,000 ml, prepare patient for an immediate thoracotomy. If bloody drainage is less than 1,000 ml, continue caring for the patient as before. Monitor drainage amount carefully. Notify the doctor immediately if drainage exceeds 500 ml within the first 3 hours.
• Draw an arterial blood sample to obtain blood gas measurements.

MEDIASTINAL SHIFT

Signs and symptoms:
• History of tension pneumothorax
• Displacement of trachea and larynx from middle toward unaffected side
• Chest assessment reveals displaced cardiac dullness, shift in apex beat, and cardiac dysrhythmias
• Neck vein distention
• Severe hypotension

Special emergency nursing considerations:
• Follow the general guidelines listed on page 52.
• Place patient on cardiac monitor.
• Prepare to assist doctor immediately with insertion of flutter valve or chest tube.

PULMONARY CONTUSION

Signs and symptoms:
• History of blunt trauma to lung (usually caused by high-velocity impact)

Special emergency nursing considerations:
• Follow the general guidelines listed on page 52.

Continued

Guide to Pulmonary Emergencies
Continued

PULMONARY CONTUSION
Continued

• Administer oxygen immediately, even if patient is asymptomatic. Hypoxemia may develop rapidly.
• Put patient in high Fowler's to help ease his breathing.
• Prepare to place patient on mechanical ventilation, if necessary.
• Draw arterial blood sample to obtain blood gas measurements.
• Prepare patient for chest X-ray.
• Place patient on cardiac monitor.
• If the patient's lost a large amount of blood, the doctor may do an emergency thoracotomy. Be prepared to assist him.

RUPTURED DIAPHRAGM

Signs and symptoms:
• History of blunt trauma (usually one-sided) or multiple trauma (especially involving fractured pelvis)
• Severe chest pain or referred pain in abdomen or shoulder; (pnea and cyanosis; chest assessment reveals decreased or absent breath sounds on affected side; and dullness, tympany, or bowel sounds on affected side from herniated viscera
• Possible mediastinal or tracheal shift away from affected side
• *Important:* In some cases, patient may be asymptomatic.

Special emergency nursing considerations:
• Follow the general guidelines listed on page 52.
• Carefully examine and evaluate entrance and exit wounds. The diaphragm's position at the time of the accident will determine the extent of injury. For example, a bullet that enters on the anterior *right* side of the patient's rib cage (above the costal margin) and exits on the posterior right side (at the 10th-rib level) will involve the patient's liver. A similar injury on the patient's *left* side will involve his spleen, stomach, colon, and small bowel.
• Administer oxygen, as ordered. Prepare to intubate patient, if necessary, and use mechanical ventilation.
• Place patient on cardiac monitor.
• Insert nasogastric tube to prevent possible respiratory and circulatory impairment from herniated abdominal viscera. If ordered, use suction or administer an iced saline solution lavage to relieve gastric bleeding.
• If the patient's lung has been punctured, get ready to assist the doctor with chest tube insertion.
• Prepare patient for surgery, if necessary.

Identifying Chest Deformities

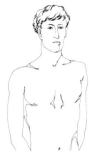

Funnel chest

Funnel chest
Physical characteristics
Sinking or funnel-shaped depression of lower sternum; diminished anteroposterior chest diameter

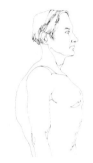

Barrel chest

CARDIOPULMONARY EMERGENCIES

Pigeon chest

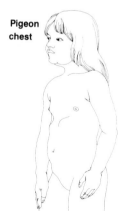

Barrel chest
Physical characteristics
Enlarged anteroposterior and transverse chest dimensions; chest appears barrel-shaped; prominent accessory muscles

Pigeon chest
Physical characteristics
Projection of sternum beyond abdomen's frontal plane. Evident in two variations: projection greatest at xiphoid process; projection greatest at or near center of sternum

Does Your Patient Have an Obstructed Airway?

Suspect airway obstruction when your patient:
• begins clutching at his throat
• suddenly loses the ability to speak
• displays exaggerated chest movements.
   To determine whether air is entering or leaving his lungs, cup your hand over the patient's nose and mouth to feel for exhaled air. Or place your ear close to his nose and mouth to listen for a rush of air while you watch for chest movement.
   Is your patient heading for a respiratory crisis? Know the signs of impending air obstruction:
• wheezing; stridor
• exaggerated chest movements, especially during inspiration
• tachycardia
• changes in skin color: cyanosis or pallor
• restlessness, agitation, fearful facial expression.
   As you know, aspirated food or foreign objects are responsible for many cases of airway obstruction. Other causes include:
• unconsciousness, causing the tongue to fall back and block the airway
• severe trauma to face, neck, or upper chest
• acute tracheal edema from smoke inhalation or from face and neck burns.
   Remember, absence of breathing doesn't always mean the patient has an airway obstruction. He may have:
• cardiopulmonary arrest
• toxic effect from anesthetic or other drug
• respiratory paralysis from a neuromuscular disease such as myasthenia gravis
• head or cervical spinal cord injury
• overoxygenation.
   Regardless of the cause, he needs immediate treatment.

Assisting with Endotracheal Intubation

The doctor may insert an endotracheal tube in your patient for short-term mechanical ventilation or airway management. You'll assist by gathering the necessary equipment and preparing your patient for the procedure. Or—if you're specially trained to perform this emergency procedure and your hospital's protocol permits—you may insert the tube yourself.

CARDIOPULMONARY
EMERGENCIES

EQUIPMENT

• Cuffed endotracheal tubes, assorted sizes

• Laryngoscope and blades

• Magill forceps

• Stylet

• 5- to 10-cc syringe

• Lubricant, water-soluble

• Xylocaine jelly or spray

• Ambu bag and mask

• Suction equipment—suction machine, suction catheters, sterile gloves, and sterile saline solution for irrigating and clearing the tubing

• Sedative and local anesthetic spray (for the conscious patient)

PROCEDURE

• Set up the mechanical ventilator.

• Explain the procedure to your patient, and sedate him if the doctor orders.

• Position the patient flat on his back with a small blanket or pillow under his head. This position brings the axis of the oropharynx, the posterior pharynx, and the trachea into alignment.

• Check the cuff on the endotracheal tube for leaks.

• As soon as the doctor's intubated your patient by passing the tube alongside the laryngoscope blades, inflate the cuff using the minimal leak technique.

Continued

Assisting with Endotracheal Intubation
Continued

PROCEDURE *Continued*

• Check tube placement by auscultating for bilateral breath sounds; observe the patient for chest expansion and feel for warm exhalations at the endotracheal tube's opening.

• Insert an oral airway or bite block.

• Secure the tube and airway with tape applied to skin treated with compound benzoin tincture.

• Suction secretions from the patient's mouth and endotracheal tube, as needed.

• Administer oxygen and/or initiate mechanical ventilation, as ordered.

POSSIBLE COMPLICATIONS

• Broken teeth

• Vocal cord damage

• Improper tube placement resulting in *esophageal intubation,* causing stomach distention or rupture from forced air pressure; or *right mainstem bronchus* intubation, so only the right lung is ventilated

• Death from asphyxia due to aspiration.

NURSING FOLLOW-UP CARE

• Suction secretions as needed, at least every 1 or 2 hours, using aseptic technique.

• Record the volume of air needed to inflate the cuff.

• *Caution:* Overinflation of the cuff can cause tracheal necrosis, so check the cuff pressure once each shift.

• Have a chest X-ray done to check tube placement.

• Restrain and reassure your patient as necessary.

• Check for adequate cuff inflation. Correct any air leaks, using the minimal leak technique.

Warning: Accidental Extubation

Any number of events may lead to endotracheal extubation. For example, a confused or disoriented patient may pull out the tube; saliva may loosen the tape anchoring the tube; or the tape may not stick well to a diaphoretic patient's skin.

Watch for the following signs and symptoms of extubation, then perform the appropriate nursing interventions. Remember that unless you intervene immediately, an extubated patient may develop progressive hypoxia, tissue damage, or acidosis—or die of asphyxiation.

CARDIOPULMONARY EMERGENCIES

EARLY WARNING SIGNS

The tube may be extubating if:
• it appears much longer than it should.
• (for a patient attached to a ventilator) the low-pressure alarm and the exhaled volume alarm (spirometer alarm) sound.
• the patient shows signs and symptoms of hypoxia: tachypnea, tachycardia, diaphoresis, anxiety, agitation, dysrhythmias, bradycardia, or cyanosis.

NURSING INTERVENTIONS

• Remove any portion of the tube that's still in place.
• Ventilate the patient using mouth-to-mouth resuscitation or an Ambu (or anesthesia) bag.
• Send someone to notify the doctor to reintubate the patient.
• Restrain the patient if he's purposely extubated himself, to prevent it from happening again.
• Each time the patient's repositioned, check the tape holding the reinserted tube.
• To make the tube secure, anchor tape from the nape of his neck to and around the tube.

Nursing Tip

Remember this: A patient being mechanically ventilated should *always* have an Ambu bag and suctioning equipment at his bedside. At the beginning of your shift, check to be sure you're prepared—if the ventilator fails, this equipment could save your patient's life.

Assisting with Emergency Cricothyroidotomy

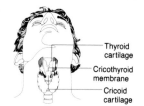

Thyroid cartilage
Cricothyroid membrane
Cricoid cartilage

Cricothyroidotomy is the opening or puncture of the trachea through the cricothyroid membrane. It's the procedure of choice when endotracheal intubation or conventional tracheotomy cannot quickly provide an airway, such as in a clinic or a doctor's office. The cricothyroid membrane may be opened with a scalpel or may be punctured with an 11G needle or a special emergency tracheotomy needle. Ideally, this is a sterile procedure. In an emergency situation outside the hospital, maintaining sterile technique may be impossible.

To assist the doctor with this procedure:

● Obtain an emergency tray containing povidone-iodine solution, sterile 4″ x 4″ gauze sponges, a scalpel, and a Delaborde dilator, or an 11G needle, or a tracheotomy needle, plus a stethoscope.

● Extend the patient's head and neck to expose the incision site and provide proper tracheal position.

● Prepare the neck with povidone-iodine solution. The doctor then locates the proper site (see illustration), makes the incision, and inserts a Delaborde dilator to prevent tissues from closing around the incision. Or he may insert an 11G needle into the cricothyroid membrane and direct the needle downward and posteriorly to avoid damaging the vocal cords. He then tapes the dilator or needle in place.

● Auscultate bilaterally for breath sounds and take vital signs.

● Once ventilation is achieved and the patient is in the hospital, blood is drawn for arterial blood gas analysis to assess the adequacy of ventilation.

● Immediately following cricothyroidotomy, watch for excessive bleeding at the insertion site, subcutaneous emphysema or inadequate ventilation from incorrect equipment placement, and tracheal or vocal cord damage. Infection may occur several days after this procedure, especially if sterile technique was compromised.

● Document the incident, including date and time, events necessitating the procedure, and the patient's vital signs. If the patient is to be transferred to an ambulance, give the attendant a verbal report.

Patricia L. Fuchs, CRTT, RRT

Comparing Artificial Airways

When a patient's threatened by an upper airway obstruction, inserting an artifical airway may be one of your first priorities. But choosing an *appropriate* airway depends on several factors, including the patient's condition. This chart details the points to consider before taking action.

OROPHARYNGEAL

Indications:
• Airway obstruction, when nasopharyngeal airway is contraindicated because of nasal obstruction or predisposition to epistaxis
• Short-term intubation

Contraindications:
• Trauma to lower face
• Oral surgery

Advantages:
• Easily inserted
• Holds tongue away from pharynx

Disadvantages:
• Dislodges easily
• May stimulate gag reflex
• May cause obstruction if airway size is incorrect
• Poorly tolerated by most conscious patients

NASOPHARYNGEAL

Indications:
• Airway obstruction, when oropharyngeal airway is contraindicated because of trauma to lower face or oral surgery
• Surgery, to maintain patent airway until patient recovers from anesthesia

Contraindications:
• Nasal obstruction
• Predisposition to epistaxis

Advantages:
• Easily inserted
• Tolerated better than oropharyngeal airway by conscious patients
• Allows for suctioning without displacing the patient's nasal turbinates

Disadvantages:
• May cause severe epistaxis if inserted too forcefully
• May kink and clog, obstructing airway
• May cause pressure necrosis of nasal mucosa
• May cause air passage obstruction, if artificial airway is too large

Continued

Comparing Artificial Airways
Continued

ORAL ESOPHAGEAL

Indications:
• Airway obstruction, when all other efforts to maintain an open airway have failed (used primarily in emergency departments or by trained paramedics)

Contraindications:
• Trauma to lower face
• Oral surgery

Advantages:
• Quickly and easily inserted
• Prevents aspiration of stomach contents while tube is in place

Disadvantages:
• May cause pharyngeal trauma during insertion
• May be accidentally inserted into trachea
• May cause gastric distension and may impair ventilation if cuff is improperly inflated

ORAL ENDOTRACHEAL

Indications:
• Cardiopulmonary resuscitation or other airway obstruction, when all other efforts to maintain an open airway have failed and when patient has nasal obstruction or predisposition to epistaxis
• Mechanical ventilation, when patient has nasal obstruction or predisposition to epistaxis
• Short-term intubation

Contraindications:
• Trauma to lower face
• Oral surgery

Advantages:
• Quickly and easily inserted
• Causes less intubation trauma than nasal endotracheal airway or trach tube
• Prevents aspiration of stomach contents, if cuff is inflated

Disadvantages:
• May damage teeth or lacerate lips, mouth, pharyngeal mucosa, or larynx during insertion
• Activates gag reflex in conscious patient
• Kinks and clogs easily
• May be bitten or chewed
• May cause pressure necrosis, middle-ear infection, laryngeal edema, or tracheal damage

Continued

Comparing Artificial Airways
Continued

NASAL ENDOTRACHEAL

Indications:
- Airway obstruction, when all other efforts to maintain an open airway have failed and when patient has facial trauma
- Mechanical ventilation
- Long-term intubation

Contraindications:
- Nasal obstruction
- Fractured nose
- Sinusitis
- Predispostion to epistaxis

Advantages:
- More comfortable than oral endotracheal tube
- Permits good oral hygiene
- Can't be bitten or chewed
- Can be anchored in place easily
- Prevents aspiration of stomach contents, if cuff is inflated

Disadvantages:
- May lacerate pharyngeal mucosa or larynx during insertion
- Kinks and clogs easily
- Increases airway resistance
- May cause pressure necrosis, middle-ear infection, laryngeal edema, or tracheal damage

TRACHEOSTOMY

Indications:
- Complete upper airway obstruction, when endotracheal intubation is impossible
- Long-term intubation

Contraindications:
- Whenever patient's highly susceptible to infection; for example, when he's receiving an immunosuppressant drug
- Short-term intubation

Advantages:
- Suctioned more easily than endotracheal tube
- Reduces dead air space in respiratory tract
- Permits patient to swallow and eat more easily
- More comfortable than other tubes
- Prevents aspiration of stomach contents, if cuff is inflated

Disadvantages:
- Requires surgery to insert
- May cause laceration or pressure necrosis of trachea
- May cause tracheoesophageal fistula
- Increases risk of tracheal and stomal inflammation, infection, and mucous plugs

Managing Status Asthmaticus

CARDIOPULMONARY
EMERGENCIES

Unless it's promptly and correctly treated, status asthmaticus may lead to fatal respiratory failure. The patient with increasingly severe asthma unresponsive to drug therapy (status asthmaticus) is usually admitted to the ICU for the following special nursing care:
• Frequently check arterial blood gas measurements to assess respiratory status, particularly after ventilator therapy or a change in oxygen concentration, or when administering $NaHCO_3$ (to correct or prevent metabolic acidosis).

• Carefully administer oxygen (the patient will be hypoxemic) and, if necessary, assist in endotracheal intubation and mechanical ventilation (when he has an elevated Pco_2).
• Administer I.V. fluids according to the patient's clinical status and age. (Dehydration is likely because of inadequate fluid intake and increased insensible loss.)
• As ordered, give corticosteroids, epinephrine, and aminophylline I.V. (Use sedation with caution.)
• Help position the patient for frequent routine chest X-rays.

What Happens in Status Asthmaticus

Status asthmaticus is a complication of asthma defined as an increasingly severe asthmatic attack that's unresponsive to bronchodilator therapy. With both nonallergic and allergic asthma, overreaction of the airways in response to irritation results in bronchoconstriction and increased mucus secretion. Simultaneous cholinergic stimulation causes the mast cells to produce the chemical mediators that lead to bronchospasm. Airway resistance and

respiratory work increase, and expiratory flow decreases, trapping air and hyperinflating alveoli. Ventilation is impaired.

Although the patient is working harder to breathe, he can't improve his oxygen supply, so he becomes hypoxic and eventually hypercapnic. As he tires, his compensatory mechanisms become less and less effective. If this process isn't reversed promptly, the patient will die.

Highlighting Aminophylline

A fine line exists between amino-phylline's therapeutic value in a patient with status asthmaticus and its toxic effects. The following guidelines will help you to administer the I.V. form of theophylline—safely.

• Find out if your patient's been taking theophylline in any form. (Keep in mind that some over-the-counter bronchodilators, such as Bronkotabs and Primatene M and P, contain theophylline.) If he has, have a serum theophylline level taken to determine his exact blood level of the drug.
• Ask the patient if he smokes cigarettes. If he does, note his age. Why? Because the age of a person who smokes affects the rate at which he metabolizes theophylline. Young adult smokers, for example, need a larger maintenance dose. Older nonsmokers—particularly those with cor pulmonale, congestive heart failure, or liver disease—need a smaller maintenance dose.
• Because a fast infusion can cause convulsions, use an I.V. infusion pump or a minidripper to administer the drug.

• If you administer aminophylline by I.V. piggyback, shut off the I.V. system already in place until the drug infuses.
• The usual loading dose is 5 to 6 mg/kg. This is followed by an infusion of 0.3 to 0.9 mg/kg/hr.
• Divide the daily dose into separate bags for infusion over 6-hour or 12-hour periods.
• Monitor the drug's effects carefully. Check your patient's pulse and blood pressure, and monitor his heartbeat for dysrhythmias. If you detect a dysrhythmia, *immediately* notify the doctor and stop the infusion.
• Aminophylline has a diuretic effect, so record your patient's intake and output to check for dehydration.
• Monitor the patient's serum theophylline levels after the first hour of administration, then after 12 and 24 hours. Therapeutic levels are between 10 and 20 mcg/ml.
• Watch for signs and symptoms of drug toxicity: anorexia, nausea, vomiting, abdominal pain, and nervousness. Notify the doctor if you detect any of these.
• Check the I.V. site frequently—the patient's breathing difficulty will make him very restless, so he may dislodge the I.V.

Anaphylaxis: Assessment and Prevention

HIGH-RISK SUBSTANCES

Antibiotics:
• penicillin and synthetic analogues, cephalosporins, tetracyclines, streptomycin, erythromycin, nitrofurantoin
Other drugs:
• aspirin, iodides, iron, dextran, tranquilizers, procaine, cocaine, benzocaine
Diagnostic agents:
• iodinated contrast media (IVP dye), Telepaque (gallbladder dye), sulfobromophthalein (BSP), sodium dehydrocholate (Decholin), Congo red
Biologicals:
• antitoxins, vaccines, gamma globulin, insulin, adrenocorticotropic hormone, enzymes
Foods:
• eggs, milk, nuts, seafood
Insect stings:
• bees, wasps, hornets, and others

SYMPTOMS

Respiratory distress:
• dyspnea, wheezing, choking, airway obstruction, cyanosis
Dermatologic changes:
• urticaria, erythema, angioedema, and pruritus
Gastrointestinal complaints:
• nausea, vomiting, abdominal cramps, diarrhea
Vascular collapse:
• rapidly falling blood pressure, sweating, weakness, anxiety, dizziness, thready pulse

Note: Symptoms may progress rapidly to cardiovascular respiratory arrest.

PREVENTION TIPS

Take a complete patient history.
Ask the patient about:
• drug allergies and the types of reactions they caused
• food, insect sting, or inhalant allergies.
Before giving any medication, **always identify the drug and ask the patient if he's ever taken it.** Never rely on a chart, cardex, bracelet, or
Continued

Anaphylaxis: Assessment and Prevention
Continued

sign to alert you to patient allergies.

If the patient had a prior reaction to the drug, have a substitute drug ordered, if possible. Otherwise, take appropriate desensitization or preventive measures, as ordered, and administer the drug slowly and cautiously.

Encourage the patient with known allergies to wear a Medic Alert bracelet or necklace. If your patient must carry an anaphylaxis kit, review the instructions with him carefully.

Always have appropriate emergency drugs/equipment on hand when administering drugs with known high anaphylaxis risk.

Remember: Even if a patient has taken a drug without incident in the past, this is no guarantee against future reactions; hypersensitivity may develop at any time.

Nursing Tip

Special Note: With a patient in anaphylactic shock, don't waste precious time trying to detect the antigen if it's not immediately apparent. Proceed at once with emergency treatment.

• Make sure your patient has an open airway.

• Administer appropriate medications.

• Monitor your patient's vital signs.

• Teach the patient how to prevent further episodes.

• Document your patient's allergy on all his records.

Five Steps for Fast Intervention

Maintain an open airway	Assess the patient's breathing. If he develops a sudden airway obstruction (from laryngeal edema), give mouth-to-mouth resuscitation, or insert an oral airway and apply mechanical ventilation. Keep an emergency tray on hand in case the doctor has to perform a tracheotomy.
Administer epinephrine	*Recommended dosage:* 0.2 to 1 ml epinephrine 1:1,000 I.M. or subcutaneously. If needed, repeat the dose four or five times at 3- to 5-minute intervals. Vigorously massage the injection site to increase absorption. Epinephrine may produce complete reversal of the patient's symptoms.
Administer an antihistamine	*Recommended dosage:* 50 to 100 mg diphenhydramine (Benadryl) P.O., I.M., or I.V., depending on patient's condition, size, and age. Giving an antihistamine with epinephrine may be the last treatment step the patient needs.
Administer fluids	If symptoms of shock continue, start an I.V. with lactated Ringer's solution, using a large-bore catheter. This will support the patient's jeopardized circulatory system. The large-bore catheter makes it easier to give medications I.V.
Check blood pressure regularly	If the patient's blood pressure drops rapidly, administer a vasopressor (such as norepinephrine) I.V. to constrict the vessels. *Recommended dosage:* 4 ml of the commercially prepared solution added to 1 liter of 5% dextrose in water. *Caution:* Watch the injection site carefully for signs of drug infiltration (redness and swelling) to prevent tissue necrosis.

Note: If the reaction's severe, the doctor may also order aminophylline to combat bronchospasms.

Important: Keep emergency drugs/equipment handy in either a crash cart or an emergency box.

Assessing Chest Wound Damage

Organs possibly affected by chest wounds

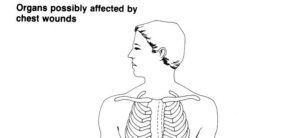

Liver
Gallbladder
Spleen
Stomach
Intestine

When assessing chest wounds, try to imagine what organs or vessels may have been damaged—based upon your knowledge of thoracic anatomy.

The scapula usually comes to the level of the seventh rib posteriorly. The dome of the diaphragm on the right usually reaches the level of the fifth rib anteriorly, and on the left to the level of the sixth rib anteriorly. The left ventricle usually lies medial to the nipple line anteriorly with the apex in the fifth intercostal space in the midclavicular line.

The apices of the lung often extend above the clavicle bilaterally, and the subclavian vessels lie closely related to the clavicle. Thus, injuries at the base of the neck may cause a pneumothorax. Anterior injuries below the level of the fifth rib on the right may affect the liver, and below the sixth rib on the left they may affect the spleen.

Managing a Sucking Chest Wound

If a sharp object or fragment from a missile injury penetrated your patient's chest wall, it may have created a sucking chest wound. Use your ears as well as your eyes to detect a sucking wound. You'll probably hear a sucking wound before you see it.

Realize, of course, that a sucking chest wound can be life-threatening. It destroys the necessary pressure gradient between the pleural space and outside atmosphere. Unless you can restore this pressure gradient, the patient may quickly develop pneumothorax, mediastinal shift, and then respiratory failure.

EQUIPMENT

• Nasal cannula, face masks, oxygen equipment
• Petrolatum gauze
• Wide tape
• Chest tube tray.

PROCEDURE

• Monitor your patient closely.
• Administer oxygen through a nasal cannula or a face mask.
• Don't remove any object protruding from your patient's chest—doing so will destroy the pressure gradient even faster and increase bleeding.

• Reassure the patient, then ask him to exhale forcefully. At the moment of maximum expiration, cover the wound with petrolatum gauze to seal it.
• Secure the gauze with wide tape.
• Monitor the patient closely for signs and symptoms of tension pneumothorax, and notify the doctor if this condition develops.
• If the doctor decides to insert a chest tube, get the equipment ready and be prepared to assist.
• If the doctor orders surgery, prepare your patient appropriately.

Chest Trauma Priorities

Order your priorities for a chest trauma patient as follows:
• Establish an open airway.
• Watch for signs of cardiac tamponade and treat it.
• Control hemorrhage.

Assisting with Chest Tube Insertion

The doctor places a chest tube in your patient's pleural space to:
• drain air, blood, fluid, or pus from his pleural space
• reestablish atmospheric and intrathoracic pressure gradients
• allow complete lung reexpansion.
   You may assist by reassuring the patient, preparing him for the procedure, and monitoring his recovery.

INDICATIONS

• Pneumothorax
• Hemothorax
• Empyema
• Pleural effusion
• Chylothorax

COMPLICATIONS

• Bleeding from intercostal blood vessels at insertion site
• Pulmonary laceration
• Tube placed into lung instead of pleural space
• Tension pneumothorax

EQUIPMENT

• Sterile gloves
• Betadine solution and prep sponges
• Sterile drapes
• Petrolatum gauze
• Dressing sponges and tape
• Local anesthetic, needles, syringes
• Chest tube tray that includes scalpel, assorted hemostats, curved clamps (Kelly), trocar, chest tubes of assorted sizes
• Underwater-seal chest drainage system (Your hospital may use the disposable Pleur-evac system, its equivalent three-bottle drainage system, or a one- or two-bottle water-seal system.)

PROCEDURE

• Explain the procedure to the patient, indicating that this procedure will help him breathe more easily.
• Sedate him as ordered.
• Assist in preparing his skin with povidone-iodine solution.
• Drape the area with sterile towels.
• The doctor will anesthetize the skin area where he plans to insert the tube.
• Help the patient hold still while the doctor makes a skin incision and inserts the tube.
                                    Continued

Assisting with Chest Tube Insertion
Continued

CARDIOPULMONARY EMERGENCIES

PROCEDURE *Continued*

• To relieve *pneumothorax*, the doctor will insert the chest tube in the second intercostal space along the midclavicular line. For *pleural effusion* or *hemothorax*, he'll insert it in the fourth to sixth intercostal space in the anterior or midaxillary line.
• Connect the tube to the Pleur-evac underwater-seal chest drainage system.
• The doctor will suture the tube in place and apply petrolatum gauze and a sterile dressing.
• Tape all tube connections securely and regulate suction as ordered.
• Secure the Pleur-evac system to the patient's bed.

NURSING FOLLOW-UP CARE

• Prepare the patient for a chest X-ray to check tube placement.
• Administer pain medication, as ordered.

• Secure the tube to the draw sheet with a safety pin, allowing sufficient tubing for the patient to turn over. Don't leave dangling loops.
• Keep clamps and extra petrolatum gauze at the patient's bedside in case the tubing accidentally disconnects or pulls out.
• Watch for signs of chest tube occlusion from kinks, clots, or mucous plugs.
• Record hourly drainage on the collection chamber of the Pleur-evac.
• Observe the suction chamber for continuous bubbling. Lack of bubbling may indicate suction failure.
• Every 2 to 4 hours, check for fluctuation on respiration in water-seal chamber: turn off the suction and observe. Fluctuation will stop when the tubing is obstructed or the lung has reexpanded. If you observe air bubbles while the suction's turned off, check the tubing for an air leak.
• Report subcutaneous emphysema, chest pressure, cyanosis, or rapid, shallow breathing to the doctor.

Initial GI Assessment Checklist
Assess the ABCs first and intervene appropriately.

CHECK FOR:

• vomiting and abdominal distention, possibly indicating bowel obstruction, peptic ulcer, or internal bleeding
• tachycardia, hypotension, diaphoresis, or pallor, possibly indicating occult bleeding and impending hypovolemia
• pain, guarding, or rigidity, indicating peritoneal irritation.

INTERVENE BY:

• establishing an I.V. and infusing fluids
• inserting a nasogastric tube.

PREPARE FOR:

• insertion of a Sengstaken-Blakemore tube
• peritoneal lavage
• emergency endoscopy
• insertion of a central venous pressure line.

ABDOMINAL/PELVIC EMERGENCIES

Seat Belt Syndrome: Watch for Hidden Abdominal Injuries

Wearing a seat belt can prevent serious injury, particularly to the head. But you need to keep in mind that using the belt improperly (wearing only the lap belt without the shoulder harness, or wearing the lap belt over the iliac crest), may *cause* injury to the abdomen.

In a car crash, abrupt deceleration compresses a passenger's seat belt into his abdomen, greatly increasing intraabdominal pressure and the pressure within hollow organs—such as his stomach and bowel. This pressure may cause rupture, laceration, or herniation of abdominal organs. In addition, shearing stress from abrupt abdominal twisting and bending may cause tissue tearing, organ transection, or vertebral injury.

So you must *always* consider the possibility of hidden abdominal injuries in a car-crash victim who was wearing a seat belt.

Guide to Abdominal/Pelvic Emergencies

LACERATED OR FRACTURED LIVER

Signs and symptoms:
● Pain in right upper abdominal quadrant
● Signs of hypovolemic shock: rapid, thready pulse; low blood pressure; anxiety; restlessness; apprehension; decreased red blood cell count; elevated white blood cell count; cool, clammy skin; pallor
● History of blunt or penetrating abdominal trauma

Special emergency nursing considerations:
● If the doctor determines the patient has a large laceration or a fractured liver, he'll want you to prepare the patient for surgery.
● If he determines the patient has a small tear, he may let it heal without further treatment.
● Be ready to administer antibiotics, tetanus toxoid, as ordered by the doctor.
● Continue to observe patient for signs and symptoms.
● Be ready to assist doctor with peritoneal lavage.

Possible associated injuries:
● Lacerated bowel
● Right lower rib fractures
● Avulsion of major hepatic vessels

RUPTURED SPLEEN

Signs and symptoms:
● Muscle spasm and rigidity in left upper abdominal quadrant
● Referred pain in left shoulder and left upper abdominal quadrant (Kehr's sign), if diaphragm's irritated
● Abdominal tenderness (in a conscious patient)
● Signs of hypovolemic shock, sometimes delayed
● Enlarged spleen with medial displacement (evident in X-ray)

Special emergency nursing considerations:
● Be ready to assist doctor with peritoneal lavage to confirm diagnosis.
● Be ready to administer antibiotics, tetanus toxoid, as ordered by the doctor.
● Prepare patient for possible arteriography.
● Prepare patient for surgery.

Possible associated injuries:
● Left lower rib fractures
● Stomach compression
● Penetrating injuries of the stomach, pancreas, and bowel (splenic flexure)

Continued

Guide to Abdominal/Pelvic Emergencies
Continued

FRACTURED PANCREAS

Signs and symptoms:
• Signs of hypovolemic shock
• Mild epigastric tenderness immediately after the injury; decreases over the next 2 hours, then worsens within 6 hours.
• Absence of bowel sounds
• Involuntary abdominal muscle spasm
• Possible elevated serum amylase
• History of blunt or penetrating abdominal trauma

Special emergency nursing considerations:
• Be ready to administer antibiotics, tetanus toxoid, as ordered by the doctor.
• Prepare patient for surgery.

Possible associated injuries:
• Crushed duodenum
• Retroperitoneal cellulitis and abscess, pancreatic pseudocyst, and chronic recurrent pancreatitis

PERFORATED GASTROINTESTINAL TRACT

Signs and symptoms:
• Lower abdominal rigidity, with spasms

• Appearance of blood in nasogastric fluid upon aspiration, possibly indicating perforated stomach
• Epigastric tenderness
• History of penetrating trauma to upper abdomen or lower thorax

Special emergency nursing considerations:
• Be ready to administer antibiotics, as ordered by the doctor.
• Prepare the patient for surgery.
• Insert a nasogastric tube for aspiration of nasogastric contents.

Possible associated injuries:
• Lacerated duodenum, jejunum, and distal ileum
• Small laceration of mesentery
• Spillage of bowel contents into peritoneal cavity, with ensuing peritonitis
• Perforated pancreas
• Intramural hematoma
• Liver or spleen injuries

LACERATED INFERIOR VENA CAVA

Signs and symptoms:
• Signs of hypovolemic shock
Note: If your patient has retroperitoneal hematoma, he may not have signs of shock.
• History of penetrating abdominal wound

Continued

ABDOMINAL/PELVIC
EMERGENCIES

Guide to Abdominal/Pelvic Emergencies
Continued

ABDOMINAL/PELVIC
EMERGENCIES

LACERATED INFERIOR VENA CAVA
Continued

Special emergency nursing considerations:
• Control severe hemorrhage; apply a MAST suit, as ordered.
• Don't start an I.V. in the patient's leg.
• Prepare patient for surgery.

Possible associated injuries:
• Lacerated abdominal aorta or bowel
• Retroperitoneal hematoma

LACERATED ABDOMINAL AORTA

Signs and symptoms:
• Abdominal tenderness and rigidity
• Signs of hypovolemic shock
• History of penetrating abdominal wound

Special emergency nursing considerations:
• Don't start an I.V. in the patient's leg, because the fluid may escape into his abdominal cavity.
• Prepare patient for immediate surgery.

Possible associated injuries:
• Lacerated inferior vena cava or bowel
• Spinal cord injury

URETHRAL TRANSECTION

Signs and symptoms:
• Gross bleeding or dried blood at urethral orifice
• Perineal ecchymosis
• Suprapubic pain
• Difficult urination, accompanied by distended bladder; urge to urinate
• Upwardly displaced prostate (in male patient)

Special emergency nursing considerations:
• Instruct patient not to urinate.
• Notify urologist.
• Be prepared to assist urologist with insertion of suprapubic catheter. *Caution:* Don't insert a Foley catheter into the urethra.
• Prepare patient for surgery.

Possible associated injuries:
• Perforated bladder
• Rectal laceration

FRACTURED PELVIS

Signs and symptoms:
• Signs of hypovolemic shock
• Pain in abdomen and back
• Absent or diminished bowel sounds
• Vomiting
• Hematuria

Continued

Guide to Abdominal/Pelvic Emergencies
Continued

FRACTURED PELVIS
Continued

• Paralytic ileus
• History of blunt abdominal/pelvic trauma

Special emergency nursing considerations:
• Be prepared to insert a nasogastric tube.
• Insert Foley catheter, as ordered by the doctor.
• Stabilize patient's pelvis with a draw sheet or pillow. If available, apply a MAST suit, as indicated by the doctor, to reduce hemorrhage and counteract hypovolemia.
• If ordered by the doctor, prepare patient for cystogram, to rule out bladder damage.
• Prepare patient for abdominal/pelvic X-rays and/or arteriography.
• Prepare patient for surgery.
• After the patient's admitted, be ready to assist doctor with application of a pelvic sling.

Possible associated injuries:
• Perforated bladder or lower bowel
• Urethral tears (more common in males)
• Displaced prostate, surrounded by a collection of blood
• Nerve damage, especially if the patient has a fractured sacrum

• Lacerated uterus
• Lacerated colon

RENAL TRAUMA

Signs and symptoms:
• Pain in midback or flank
• Referred abdominal pain, which may worsen with movement
• Hematuria (may be frank or occult)
• Oliguria or anuria
• Local ecchymosis, with possible edema
• Local tenderness to the touch
• History of penetrating thoracic, abdominal, or lower back trauma

Special emergency nursing considerations:
• Insert a Foley catheter.
• Be prepared to assist with a bladder irrigation.
• Apply ice packs to reduce swelling.
• Prepare patient for a possible cystogram, intravenous pyelogram (IVP), or renal arteriography, as ordered by the doctor.
• After diagnostic tests are performed, administer analgesics, as ordered by the doctor.
• In cases of severe trauma, prepare patient for surgery.

Possible associated injury:
• Fractured pelvis

Continued

ABDOMINAL/PELVIC
EMERGENCIES

Guide to Abdominal/Pelvic Emergencies
Continued

PERFORATED BLADDER

Signs and symptoms:
• Pain in lower abdominal or suprapubic area
• Signs of hypovolemic shock
• Difficulty with bowel movement,
accompanied by urge to void
• Hematuria
• Ecchymosis or bruising on
lower abdomen, below the umbilicus
• Large, suprapubic mass (possibly from a perivesical collection of
urine and blood)

Special emergency nursing considerations:
• Insert a Foley catheter to obtain
urine specimen.
• If urethral damage accompanies
the bladder trauma, be prepared
to assist the doctor with insertion
of suprapubic catheter.
• Prepare patient for a cystogram
or an IVP, as ordered by the doctor.
• Prepare patient for immediate
surgery.

Possible associated injuries:
• Perforated peritoneum
• Urethral damage

Tracing Trajectories

To determine the extent of internal damage in cases of abdominal penetration wounds,
try estimating the missile's
trajectory. Consider its magni-
tude and whether it was applied directly or indirectly.

If your patient has a *penetrating injury*, you can commonly expect less secondary
trauma than if he has a blunt
injury, because a penetrating
injury usually involves less
energy. Stab wounds, in particular, are relatively low-en-

ergy wounds, which may involve only one or two body
systems.

Evaluate the entrance and
exit wounds and then gauge
what organs lie in the path
between them. In cases of
stab wounds, note the angle
of the weapon but don't try to
remove it yourself. Assess the
patient's condition as rapidly
and accurately as possible,
and then have him prepared
for surgery.

Eight Trouble Indicators: What They Suggest

Any of the following conditions in a patient with an abdominal/pelvic injury may indicate a serious—perhaps life-threatening—situation. Notify the doctor at once.

SIGN	WHAT IT SUGGESTS
KEHR'S: Referred pain at tip of left shoulder and in left upper quadrant	Ruptured spleen or diaphragmatic irritation from blood, bile, or fecal material
BRUIT: Abnormal sound or murmur along middle or lower back	Arterial injury, possibly of renal vascular network
BALLANCE'S: Fixed area of dullness when left upper abdominal quadrant is percussed	Subcapsular or extracapsular hematoma of spleen
TURNER'S: Bluish color on flank	Blood collecting in abdomen from fractured pancreas
CULLEN'S: Purplish color around umbilicus	Blood collecting in abdomen from fractured pancreas or ruptured ectopic pregnancy
HEMATOMA: At lumbar spine level	Internal hemorrhage, probably from fractured pelvis or fractured vertebrae
DECREASED PERISTALTIC SOUNDS: About one per minute	Paralytic ileus
COOPERNAIL: Ecchymosis on scrotum or labia	Fractured pelvis

ABDOMINAL/PELVIC EMERGENCIES

Assessing the Acute Abdomen

TEST/PROCEDURE	IMPLICATIONS OF FINDINGS
HYPERESTHESIA TEST Using the point of a pin, gently stroke the abdomen of the supine patient from the upper to the lower areas.	Sharper sensation at any location suggests visceral or parietal peritoneal irritation.
REBOUND TENDERNESS With the patient supine, apply deep pressure to the abdomen away from the suspected site of inflammation. Then quickly release pressure.	Pain felt upon release of pressure indicates peritoneal irritation. It may be localized or general.
MURPHY'S SIGN As the supine patient takes a deep breath, perform deep palpation in the right upper quadrant, making contact with the gallbladder	Sharp pain and arrested inspiration suggest cholecystitis.
ILIOPSOAS TEST Instruct the supine patient to flex the right hip against moderate resistance over the thigh. Or position the patient on his left side, and have him flex his right leg at the hip.	Pain in the right lower quadrant during psoas muscle contraction suggests an inflamed or perforated appendix.
OBTURATOR TEST Ask the supine patient to flex his right hip and knee to 90°. Rotate his ankle internally and externally.	Pain in the hypogastric area with obturator muscle involvement suggests a perforated appendix or pelvic abscess.

ABDOMINAL/PELVIC
EMERGENCIES

Danger: Peritonitis

Peritonitis—a potentially life-threatening inflammation of the visceral and parietal peritoneum—results from bacterial infection or chemical irritation that occurs when a perforated abdominal organ leaks fluid and blood into the abdominal cavity. Common causes of peritonitis are ruptured diverticuli, ruptured appendix, and penetrating abdominal trauma. But suspect it in *any* patient who has a GI disorder or a history of abdominal trauma, or who's had surgery of the abdominal cavity.

SIGNS AND SYMPTOMS

- Sudden abdominal *pain,* which may be localized or diffuse but is most intense in the area of the patient's primary GI disorder
- Abdominal *distention* and rebound *tenderness*
- Increased *temperature* (103° F., or 39.4° C.—or higher), with *chills*
- Signs of *shock* (weakness, pallor, diaphoresis, tachycardia, decreased blood pressure)
- Shallow, rapid *respirations* (due to diaphragmatic irritation).

If you note any of these signs and symptoms, notify the doctor *immediately.* Remember, peritonitis can develop very rapidly.

DIAGNOSIS

The doctor will order a complete blood count to determine if the white blood cell count is elevated. He'll also order abdominal X-rays, which may show a paralytic ileus, edema, distention of the bowels, and upward displacement of the diaphragm. He may also perform

a paracentesis to check for bacteria, exudate, pus, blood, or urine in the patient's abdominal cavity.

TREATMENT

Peritonitis is treated in three steps:
- The underlying cause is identified and treated.
- The infection is treated.
- Dehydration and paralytic ileus are corrected.

Your patient may need surgery to remove or seal off the source of peritoneal contamination, or he may have an incision and drainage if the infection is localized.

NURSING INTERVENTIONS

Expect to start antibiotics promptly. Start an I.V. for fluid and electrolyte replacement, and insert a nasogastric tube, as ordered, to aspirate stomach contents. Give the patient nothing by mouth until his bowel sounds return and his gastric aspirate becomes scanty. Administer analgesics, as ordered.

ABDOMINAL/PELVIC EMERGENCIES

Recognizing Hepatic Coma

Patients in hepatic coma progress through the following four stages, with accompanying clinical features:
• **Prodromal:** mild confusion, euphoria or depression, vacant stare, inappropriate laughter, forgetfulness, inability to concentrate, slow mentation, slurred speech, untidiness, lethargy, belligerence, minimal asterixis (flapping tremor).

Watch carefully for these subtle symptoms. They're not necessarily present at the same time.
• **Impending:** obvious obtundation, aberrant behavior, definite asterixis, constructional apraxia.

To test for asterixis (flapping tremor), have the patient raise both arms, with forearms flexed and fingers extended. To test for

constructional apraxia, keep a serial record of the patient's handwriting and figure construction, and check it for progressive deterioration.
• **Stuporous** (patient can still be aroused): marked confusion, incoherent speech, asterixis, noisiness, abusiveness, violence, abnormal EEG.

Restraints may be necessary at this stage. *Do not sedate the patient; sedation could be fatal.*
• **Comatose** (patient can't be aroused, responds only to painful stimuli): no asterixis but positive Babinski's sign, hepatic fetor (breath has musty, sweet odor), and *elevated serum ammonia level.*

Degree of hepatic fetor correlates with the degree of somnolence and confusion.

Nursing Tip

D.T. Alert: Watch for these signs and symptoms of impending DTs in *any* patient suspected of abusing alcohol:
• tremors
• agitation, confusion, and disorientation
• elevated vital signs
• signs of autonomic nervous system disorder (dilated pupils, fever, tachycardia).

If you see any of these signs and symptoms, intervene immediately. Notify the doctor, and prepare to administer tranquilizers as ordered. Try to calm your patient by creating a quiet, nonstressful atmosphere and by reassuring him in a soothing tone of voice.

Eliciting Signs and Symptoms of Appendicitis

The signs and symptoms of appendicitis are often confusingly similar to those of other illnesses, such as gastritis, colitis, and diverticulitis. To help you differentiate appendicitis from other disorders, here are four characteristic signs to look for when examining your patient:

MCBURNEY'S SIGN
Rebound tenderness and sharp pain occurring in the area of the patient's appendix when you palpate *McBurney's point,* located about 2″ (5.1 cm) below the right anterior superior spine of the ilium, on a line between the spine and the umbilicus

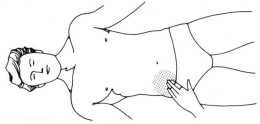

AARON'S SIGN
Pain or distress occurring in the area of the patient's heart or stomach when you palpate McBurney's point

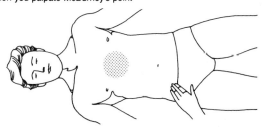

Continued

Eliciting Signs and Symptoms of Appendicitis
Continued

ROVSING'S SIGN
Pain in the patient's right lower quadrant when you apply pressure in the left lower quadrant

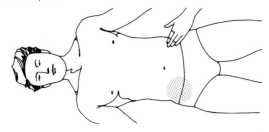

PSOAS SIGN
Increasing pain occurring in the patient's abdomen when he extends his right leg while lying on his left side, or when he flexes his legs while supine

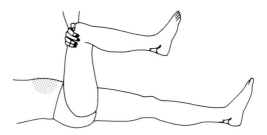

What to Do First

Your immediate assessment of a GI bleeder should cover these points:
• **_Determine if the patient's in shock._** Even if he's not, he'll need an I.V. line to provide access to circulation and for rapid fluid replacement to restore blood volume.
• **_Assess blood loss._** Hypovolemic shock doesn't begin until the patient has lost 20% of his fluid volume. Estimate the amount of blood lost by the degree of shock.
• **_Check pulse and blood pressure,_** the most important vital signs in shock, every 15 minutes until the patient's condition stabilizes.
• **_Determine if he's still vomiting blood._** He may need a nasogastric tube passed to assess the rate of bleeding and to clear the stomach for possible endoscopy. In some cases, ice lavage may be used to control the bleeding.
• **_Evaluate skin quality._** If his skin is cool and clammy, he'll probably need oxygen to improve tissue perfusion.
• **_Get a blood type and cross match,_** along with a hemoglobin and hematocrit determination. Be ready to give transfusions as the patient needs them.

ABDOMINAL/PELVIC
EMERGENCIES

Using the Tilt Test to Evaluate Hypovolemia

To measure your patient's orthostatic vital signs, take his blood pressure and pulse rate when he's in three different postures: supine, sitting, and standing. (If you note significant changes when the patient sits up, _do not_ have him stand up.)

Consider a decrease of 10 mm Hg or more in systolic pressure or an increase of 10 beats per minute or more in pulse rate as a sign of volume depletion and possible impending hypovolemic shock.

Using Color to Identify Bleeding Site

When blood is vomited or aspirated by nasogastric tube, the stomach or duodenum is almost always the site of bleeding. If the blood is bright red, it's fresh. But if it's dark red or looks like coffee grounds, it's been in contact with gastric acid for perhaps several hours.

Blood in the stool may occur alone or in association with hematemesis. The color of this blood and the stool can help pinpoint the bleeding site.

ABDOMINAL/PELVIC
EMERGENCIES

• Bright red blood only: bleeding in rectum and lower sigmoid

• Bright red blood mixed with stool: bleeding below midtransverse colon

• Bright red blood on stool surface: bleeding in rectum and lower sigmoid

• Maroon blood with diarrhea: bleeding above mid-transverse colon

• Melena with diarrhea: bleeding above ligament of Treitz

• Melena without diarrhea: bleeding above mid-transverse colon

• Blood and stool mixed with pus: bleeding caused by inflammatory disease of the colon

• Occult blood: bleeding anywhere in GI or upper respiratory tract

Highlighting Vasopressin (Pitressin)

You may be asked to administer vasopressin (Pitressin) as an adjunct to more conventional treatment for acute GI hemorrhage, such as use of the Sengstaken-Blakemore tube. Administered intravenously or intraarterially, vasopressin causes vasoconstriction that results in decreased blood flow, decreased portal pressure, and increased clotting and hemostasis. This action makes vasopressin particularly effective in the treatment of conditions precipitated by portal hypertension, such as ruptured esophageal varices.

Such treatment generally consists of an initial I.V. bolus of aqueous vasopressin for 5 to 30 minutes, with continuous I.V. infusion until 24 hours after the bleeding has stopped. While administering vasopressin, monitor your patient's heart rate, blood pressure, EKG, and renal function. Possible adverse effects include:

- decreased heart rate and cardiac output
- increased blood pressure
- abdominal cramping
- bowel infarction
- water intoxication.

Warning: When preparing vasopressin for administration, read the label carefully—different commercial products have confusingly similar names.

- Pitocin: oxytocin
- Pitressin: synthetic vasopressin
- Pitressin Tannate in Oil: vasopressin in oil diluent
- Pituitrin: posterior pituitary (vasopressin and oxytocin).

Nursing Tip

Some Causes of Lower GI Bleeding
- ulcerative colitis
- diverticulosis
- fistulas
- cecal ulcers
- tumors
- angiodysplasia
- infarcted bowel.

ABDOMINAL/PELVIC EMERGENCIES

Comparing Gastrointestinal Tubes

In an emergency, you may assist with the insertion of a GI tube to treat a patient's bowel obstruction, to aspirate his gastric or bowel contents, or to lavage his stomach. These are some of the tubes you may use. Be sure you're familiar with all of them.

GASTRIC TUBES

Levin tube

This is a 50″ (127-cm), single-lumen, rubber or plastic tube with holes at the tip and along the side. It's used to remove stomach fluid and gas or to aspirate gastric contents. It may also be used for gastric lavage, drug administration, or feeding.

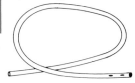

Ewald tube

A wide-bore tube that passes a large volume of fluid quickly, it's used for stomach lavage in patients who've ingested poison or who have profuse GI bleeding.

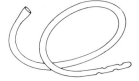

Salem-Sump tube

This 48″ (122-cm), double-lumen tube has a small air-vent lumen and a primary suction-drainage lumen. The air-vent lumen allows atmospheric air to enter the patient's stomach so the tube can float freely. This prevents the tube from adhering to the gastric mucosa and damaging it. This tube is used for the same purposes as the Levin tube.

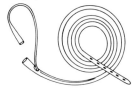

Nursing considerations:

• Attach tube to low continuous or intermittent suction, or to straight gravity drainage, as ordered.
• Before instilling anything through the tube, always verify its placement by aspirating gastric contents or by auscultating the patient's stomach while injecting 50 cc of air into the tube. (A gurgling sound means the tube's in place.)
• To maintain patency, irrigate tube with 30 cc of normal saline solution every 2 hours or as ordered.

Continued

Comparing Gastrointestinal Tubes
Continued

INTESTINAL TUBES

Miller-Abbott tube
This 10′ (3-m), double-lumen tube has one lumen for balloon inflation and one for drainage or suction. It's used in patients with bowel obstruction because it permits aspiration of bowel contents.

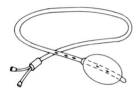

Harris tube
This 6′ (1.8-m), single-lumen tube has a metal tip and a balloon for mercury injection. Also used in patients with bowel obstruction, it permits intestinal tract lavage, usually with a Y tube attached.

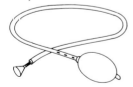

Cantor tube
This 10′ (3-m), single-lumen tube has a balloon at its distal tip for mercury injection. It's also used in patients with bowel obstruction because it permits aspiration of bowel contents.

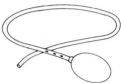

Nursing considerations:
• When using a *Miller-Abbott tube*, fill the balloon with mercury when the tube reaches the stomach, and clamp the balloon lumen to prevent accidental mercury withdrawal through suction. Label each lumen. With a *Cantor* or *Harris tube*, fill the balloon bag's upper portion with mercury before insertion, and aspirate all air from the bag.
• Place the patient on his right side for tube advancement.
• Drain the tube by gravity during insertion. If drainage stops, inject 10 cc of air.
• Confirm tube placement by X-ray.
• Attach the suction lumen to intermittent low suction when the tube reaches its mark (as ordered).

Initial Ob/Gyn Assessment Checklist

Assess the ABCs first and intervene appropriately.

ABDOMINAL/PELVIC EMERGENCIES

CHECK FOR:

• tachycardia; cool, clammy, pale skin; restlessness, indicating occult bleeding and shock
• fetal bradycardia or tachycardia, indicating fetal distress
• hypertension, edema of face and hands, proteinuria, apprehension, and vertigo, indicating preeclampsia
• generalized edema, tonic-clonic convulsions, and coma, indicating eclampsia

INTERVENE BY:

• starting an I.V. with a large-bore catheter

• administering oxygen by mask or nasal cannula
• placing the patient on her left side or in a supine position, if needed
• sending blood to the laboratory for typing and cross matching, coagulation times, and indirect Coombs' test

PREPARE FOR:

• blood transfusions
• RhoGam administration
• magnesium sulfate administration
• emergency delivery
• surgery

Nursing Tip

Determining Due Dates: Whatever the nature of your pregnant patient's emergency, you need to know her estimated date of confinement (EDC), or "due date." If she doesn't know this date, you can approximate it using a technique known as Nägele's rule:

Ask her the starting date of her last menstrual period (LMP). Subtract 3 months from this date, then add 7 days. For example, if her LMP started March 13, subtract 3 months (December 13) and add 7 days—for a December 20 EDC.

Caring for the Rape Victim

When dealing with a victim of rape, you can reduce both the trauma and her anxiety by providing effective nursing and psychological care. Follow these guidelines:

• As a first consideration, your hospital should entrust the rape victim only to the care of a nurse and doctor of the same sex as the patient (who's usually female). Place the patient in a treatment area that's quiet, private, and secure. Introduce yourself. Show acceptance for her through eye contact, tone of voice, and (if appropriate) physical contact. Your hospital may have an arrangement with a local rape crisis center. If it does, ask your patient if she'd like to have a rape victim advocate with her during her hospital stay. If your hospital doesn't have such an arrangement, assure the patient that you'll be with her at all times throughout her emergency care.

• Set priorities according to your patient's needs. Physical injuries require immediate attention.

• Don't allow her to drink fluids or to wash her genital area. Explain that such activities would remove any existing semen, which is vital medicolegal evidence.

• After the patient is reasonably calm, explain that the doctor will ask her questions to identify the type of assault made on her. Be open to discussing her feelings and her fears. Demonstrate a nonjudgmental and supportive attitude. You'll find most rape victims have a need to talk.

• Introduce all hospital personnel entering the examination area to the patient.

• Tell the patient what treatment she'll receive: the doctor will perform a head-to-toe physical examination for signs of physical trauma and may order a Pap smear of her vagina, mouth, or rectum; saline suspensions to test for sperm presence; and an acid phosphatase test to determine how recently intercourse took

Continued

Caring for the Rape Victim
Continued

place. The doctor will also order prophylactic antibiotics for sexually transmitted diseases. (When the patient is calm, discuss postcoital contraception and possible pregnancy with her.) The police will probably request the patient's articles of clothing as evidence (don't wash or discard them); they may ask you to try to find samples of the assailant's hair and skin tissue by combing the patient's pubic hair and examining her fingernails for deposits. Write down explanations of these procedures and the doctor's orders regarding such things as how often the patient should take antibiotics and when she should be reexamined. She can refer to these later.

• After your patient has been examined and treated, provide her with facilities to wash herself. Also provide mouthwash or a change of clothing, if needed. Before she leaves the hospital, be sure she understands the importance of getting retested for sexually transmitted disease in about 3 weeks, or sooner if symptoms occur. Some patients may require psychiatric referral. Give the rape victim written information about where to go for social, legal, or medical help, if needed.

Pregnancy Prophylaxis

After a rape, tell a patient about her risk of becoming pregnant. You'll need her signed consent before you give the first dose of pregnancy prophylaxis (diethylstilbestrol [DES] or another estrogen, which many women call the "morning-after pill"). The doctor should explain the risks. If your patient is too upset to decide about taking DES, tell her she has time to decide. If she decides to wait, discuss her options:

• She can make up her mind, any time within 24 hours after the attack, to start taking DES.

• She can wait to find out whether she's pregnant. If she learns she is pregnant, she can decide whether to have an abortion, to keep the child, or to put it up for adoption.

Collection of Rape Evidence

Rape generally refers to sexual intercourse between a man and a woman without the woman's consent.

To care for the rape victim:

• Take her to a private room and provide support. Offer to contact her family or friends.

• Explain the procedure and answer the patient's questions. Ask her to sign a consent form to *authorize the physical examination, collection of evidence, and treatment.* Obtain her medical history and a description of the rape.

• After the doctor performs a thorough physical examination, help him photograph the patient's injuries. *Photographs are legally admissible in court and offer proof of injury after healing has taken place.*

• Darken the room and examine the patient's clothing and body with the Wood's light. *The ultraviolet rays cause seminal fluid to appear fluorescent blue because of its high acid phosphatase levels.* Circle clothing stains that are Wood's light-positive with a laundry marker.

• Using a clean tongue blade, scrape areas that are Wood's light-positive. *Analysis of the scrapings for acid phosphatase and ABH antigen verifies the presence of semen and helps identify the assailant.*

• Comb the pubic hair *to dislodge any loose hair and foreign material.* Next, cut a few of the patient's pubic hairs. *Loose hair can be cross matched against the patient's pubic hair and that of her alleged assailant.*

• Collect clippings from each fingernail. *Skin cells or dried blood found under nails may match those of the assailant. Fibers from clothing or other material may match evidence found at the scene.*

• Collect venous blood samples—one for RPR, a test for syphilis; one for blood type and Rh factor; and one for a pregnancy test. *The patient's blood type and Rh factor must be compared to the alleged assailant's blood type, identified through nail clippings or semen analysis.*

Continued

Collection of Rape Evidence
Continued

• Before the pelvic exam, instruct the patient to urinate. Tell her not to wipe the vulva *to avoid removal of any semen.*

• If the patient has inserted a tampon, ask her to remove it; then wrap and label it.

• Place the patient in the lithotomy position and drape her. The doctor examines the external genitalia for injuries and evaluates the state of the hymen.

• The doctor inserts a lubricated speculum and inspects the cervix and vagina for trauma. *The speculum is lubricated with water because commercial lubricants retard sperm motility and interfere with specimen collection and analysis.*

• Using a cotton-tipped applicator, the doctor obtains a specimen from the posterior fornix, smears the specimen on a microscope slide, adds a drop of normal saline solution, and places a coverslip over it. *Discovery of motile sperm on this wet mount verifies sexual intercourse within the past 28 hours.*

• The doctor obtains another specimen from the posterior fornix and smears it on a slide. *Gram's stain is applied to this smear to help identify sperm.*

• The doctor collects two final specimens from the posterior fornix and places each into a test tube with normal saline solution—one to be tested for acid phosphatase, the other for ABH antigen. Store these tubes on ice until they're taken to the laboratory. The acid phosphatase test helps determine the time of the assault, *because a fresh ejaculate (from within the past 12 hours) contains the highest concentration of acid phosphatase. It also verifies the presence of seminal fluid when sperm are absent.* Like other body fluids, semen contains the soluble A, B, and H blood group substances in the 80% of males who are genetic secretors. Thus, blood group A substance in the seminal fluid points to an assailant who is a secretor with blood group A.

• The doctor collects endocervical and urethral specimens for gonorrhea culture, as well as
Continued

Collection of Rape Evidence
Continued

gonorrhea culture, as well as oral and rectal specimens, if necessary. Because collection of an endocervical specimen may dislodge motile sperm from the endocervix, this procedure must follow collection of posterior fornix secretions *to avoid collection of sperm from someone other than the assailant.*

• Carefully label all specimens, and list them in your notes.

• The doctor performs a bimanual examination of the uterus. He also examines the anus if the patient reports penetration there. After this exam, the doctor cleans any cuts and treats lacerations.

• Collect a specimen of the patient's saliva and place it in a test tube filled with normal saline solution. *An ABH antigen test of sputum determines the patient's secretory status, which is compared to that of the alleged assailant.*

• Allow the patient to wash and dress.

• Develop a follow-up care plan to meet the patient's needs. Give her the names and phone numbers of local organizations for counseling rape victims, such as Women Organized Against Rape (WOAR).

ABDOMINAL/PELVIC EMERGENCIES

Nursing Tip

Special consideration: If the rape victim is a child, realize that a young child will place only as much importance on an experience as others do unless there is physical pain. A good question to ask is, "Did someone touch you when or where you didn't want to be touched?" As with other rape victims, record information in the child's own words.

Initial Genitourinary Assessment Checklist

Assess the ABCs first and intervene appropriately.

CHECK FOR:

• ecchymoses in the flank area, indicating retroperitoneal bleeding
• a suprapubic mass or perineal mass, indicating urine extravasation
• severe, colicky flank pain, indicating renal calculi

INTERVENE BY:

• checking the patient's urine for blood with a urine testing strip, straining it for kidney stones, and sending the specimen to the laboratory for urinalysis and culture-and-sensitivity testing

• starting I.V. fluids to maintain the patient's fluid volume and to provide access to blood, if needed
• giving narcotics and analgesics, as ordered, to control pain

PREPARE FOR:

• intravenous pyelography
• a retrograde urethrogram
• suprapubic catheter insertion
• transfer of the patient to a re-plantation center

Drugs That Can Cause Hematuria

When your patient voids red or orange urine, you should tell his doctor you suspect hematuria and possible genitourinary problems, right? Not necessarily. Certain foods, drugs, and diseases can cause pseudohematuria, which looks like hematuria but is simply reddish urine with no detectable hemoglobin or blood cells. So your first move should be to check your patient's chart for pseu-dohematuria-inducing drugs he may be taking. (Examples include phenazopyridine, phenolphthalein, phenolsulfon-phthalein dye, senna, or cascara sagrada.) Then ask him what he's been eating lately—any beets, rhubarb, or blackberries? (Vegetable dyes used to color food also cause pseudohematuria.) Does he have a history of porphyria, which can also redden his urine?

Initial Neurologic Assessment Checklist

Assess the ABCs first and intervene appropriately.

CHECK FOR:	INTERVENE BY:
• change in level of consciousness, which is often the first sign of neurologic deterioration	• stabilizing the cervical spine until fracture's ruled out

PREPARE FOR:

• bradycardia and widened pulse pressure, possibly indicating increased intracranial pressure (ICP)

• lumbar puncture

• administration of osmotic diuretics

• pupillary changes, possibly indicating increased ICP, brain stem injury, or cranial nerve damage

• transportation to X-ray for computerized tomography scan

• paralysis or paresis, possibly indicating brain or spinal cord injury

NEUROLOGIC
EMERGENCIES

Making the Most of Your Neurocheck

• When performing a neurocheck, describe your observations specifically and completely.
• If you note a change in your patient's neurologic status, increase the frequency of your neuro-

checks until his condition is stable.
• At the end of your shift, ask a co-worker from the next shift to assist you with a neurocheck. Doing so helps ensure neurocheck continuity and consistency.

Assessing Level of Consciousness Using the Glasgow Coma Scale

To assess and monitor the level of consciousness of a patient with suspected or confirmed brain injury quickly, use the Glasgow Coma Scale. You'll find this scale useful in the emergency department, at the scene of an accident, and for periodic evaluation of the hospitalized patient. The Glasgow scale measures three faculties' responses to stimuli—eye opening, motor response, and verbal response. Below you'll find an expanded version of this useful—though not comprehensive—assessment technique. (The lowest a patient can score is 3, the highest 15. A patient scoring 7 or less is comatose and probably has severe neurologic damage.)

TEST/SCORE	PATIENT'S RESPONSE

Verbal response (when you ask, "What year is this?")

Oriented	5	He tells you the current year.
Confused	4	He tells you an incorrect year.
Inappropriate words	3	He replies randomly: "tomorrow" or "roses."
Incomprehensible	2	He moans or screams.
None	1	He gives no response.

Eye opening response

Spontaneously	4	He opens his eyes spontaneously.
To speech	3	He opens his eyes when you tell him to.
To pain	2	He opens his eyes only on painful stimulus (for example, application of pressure to bony ridge under eyebrow).
None	1	He doesn't open his eyes in response to any stimulus.

Continued

NEUROLOGIC
EMERGENCIES

Assessing Level of Consciousness Using the Glasgow Coma Scale
Continued

TEST/SCORE	PATIENT'S RESPONSE

Motor response

Obeys 6

He shows you two fingers when you ask him to.

Localizes 5

He reaches toward the painful stimulus and tries to remove it.

Withdraws 4

He moves away from a painful stimulus.

Abnormal flexion 3

He assumes a decorticate posture (below).

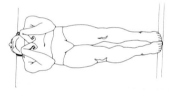

Abnormal extension 2

He assumes a decerebrate posture (below).

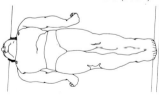

None 1

He doesn't respond at all, just lies flaccid—an *ominous sign.*

Understanding Pupillary Changes

PUPIL DESCRIPTION	POSSIBLE CAUSES
Dilated, unilateral, fixed, no reaction to light	• Uncal herniation with oculomotor nerve damage • Brain stem compression due to an expanding mass lesion or an aneurysm • Increased intracranial pressure • Tentorial herniation • Head trauma with subsequent subdural or epidural hematoma
Dilated, bilateral, fixed, no reaction to light	• Severe midbrain damage • Cardiopulmonary arrest (hypoxia) • Anticholinergic poisoning
Midsized, bilateral, fixed, no reaction to light	• Midbrain involvement due to edema, hemorrhage, infarctions, lacerations, contusions
Pinpoint, usually bilateral, no reaction to light	• Lesion of pons, usually after hemorrhage, leading to blocked sympathetic impulses • Opiates (morphine)—pupils may be reactive
Small, unilateral, no reaction to light	• Disruption of sympathetic nerve supply to head due to spinal cord lesion above T1

Assessing Extraocular Muscle Function

Test your patient's extraocular muscle function if he's suffered facial or eye trauma or has a suspected neurologic deficit. If any of the six extraocular muscles or three pairs of cranial nerves (III, IV, and VI) that control eyeball movements is impaired (because of edema, orbital fracture, or impingement), he'll have improper eye alignment, impaired eye movement, and diplopia. Here's how to check for impaired extraocular muscle function:

First, check your patient's corneal light reflex by shining a penlight directly between his eyes, holding it 12″ to 15″ (30.5 to 38.1 cm) away. You'll see a small dot of light at the same spot on each cornea, equidistant from his nose. If the dots are asymmetrical, suspect muscle impairment.

Next, check specific muscle and nerve function. Ask your patient to follow your finger (or a pencil) with his eyes as you trace the six cardinal fields of gaze in front of his face. Stop at each field and observe your patient's eyes. If both eyes don't deviate fully into each field of gaze, suspect muscle entrapment or paralysis, with possible nerve damage.

SIX CARDINAL FIELDS OF GAZE	CORRESPONDING MUSCLE
Straight nasal	Medial rectus (MR)
Up and nasal	Inferior oblique (IO)
Down and nasal	Superior oblique (SO)
Straight temporal	Lateral rectus (LR)
Up and temporal	Superior rectus (SR)
Down and temporal	Inferior rectus (IR)

NEUROLOGIC
EMERGENCIES

Danger: Increasing Intracranial Pressure

Your patient may show signs of increasing intracranial pressure (ICP) from any of the following conditions: intracranial hemorrhage, brain tumor, meningitis, or cerebral edema. Unless the condition is reversed, the patient's brain tissue will herniate through the tentorial notch, causing brain stem compression.

To ensure prompt treatment, watch your patient closely for these danger signs:
• headache complaint (an early warning sign)
• decreasing level of consciousness
• vomiting
• change in pupil size or equality, papilledema, and extraocular movements. Remember, papilledema usually takes 12 to 24 hours to develop.
• rising blood pressure, slowing pulse, hyperthermia, and a change in respiration pattern (in later stage of ICP).

If you observe any of the above, notify the doctor at once. Document your findings in your nurses' notes.

Positioning the Head-Injured Patient

As soon as you rule out or stabilize a cervical injury, put the head-injured patient in the correct position. To perform a quick assessment or deliver cardiopulmonary resuscitation, you may want to place a head-injured patient on his back; otherwise, put him far over on either side or on his abdomen in a swimmer's position. This prevents his tongue from occluding his airway and allows natural drainage of secretions. Remember, if you notice spinal fluid leaking from his nose or ears, keep his head raised 30°. *Caution:* Whenever you care for a patient with a head injury, never place his head lower than the rest of his body. In a case of hypovolemic shock, let his head stay elevated and raise his limbs as much as possible to increase venous return to the heart.

NEUROLOGIC
EMERGENCIES

Two Quick Tests for Possible Meningitis

When you suspect your patient may have meningitis, perform these two quick tests. Positive Brudzinski's and Kernig's signs—in the presence of such signs and symptoms as fever, chills, headache, stiff neck, and altered behavior and level of consciousness—indicate possible meningitis. Here's how to test your patient for Brudzinski's and Kernig's signs:

BRUDZINSKI'S SIGN

Place your patient in the dorsal recumbent position, putting your hands behind her neck and bending the neck forward. The sign's *positive* if pain and resistance are present and if the patient flexes her hips and knees in response to the maneuver.

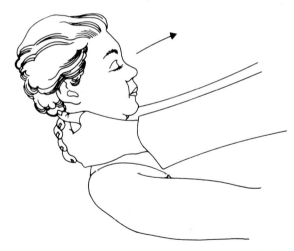

Continued

Two Quick Tests for Possible Meningitis
Continued

KERNIG'S SIGN

With your patient supine, flex her leg at the hip and knee, then try to straighten her knee. The sign's *positive* if pain and resistance are present.

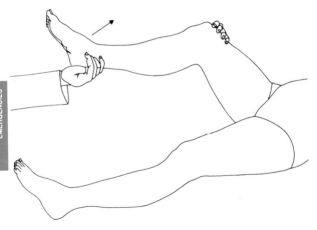

Signs and Symptoms in Head Injuries

CONCUSSION

Injury is functional:
Mild:
• transient loss of consciousness
• possible impairment of higher mental functions, such as retrograde amnesia and emotional lability
Severe:
• prolonged unconsciousness
• impairment of functions of brain stem, such as transient loss of respiratory reflex, vasomotor activity, and dilation of pupils

LACERATION (tearing of neural tissue)

Injury is organic:
• prolonged loss of consciousness
• lingering neurological deficit
• frequent involvement of frontal and temporal cortices and midbrain
• shock, headache, and vertigo in varying degrees
• convulsions and focal damage such as monoplegia or hemiplegia possible
• blood in spinal fluid

NEUROLOGIC EMERGENCIES

Highlighting Mannitol

Mannitol is an osmotic diuretic often used to decrease intracranial pressure in patients with neurologic disorders. Remember these important points when using mannitol:
• It may crystallize out of solution at concentrations of 15% or greater, especially when exposed to low temperatures. If this happens, you can warm the solution in hot water and shake it vigorously, or you can autoclave it. Be sure it's cooled to body temperature before you administer it to your patient.
• Don't use mannitol if it's not completely dissolved.
• Always administer mannitol solutions intravenously, through an in-line filter.
• Adding electrolytes to a 20% or greater solution of mannitol may cause precipitation.
• Don't infuse mannitol in the same line as whole blood; precipitation will result.

Guide to Head Injuries

A head injury can have grave, even life-threatening consequences; for example, irreversible brain or spinal damage. To prevent complications, proper emergency care is essential. Read the guidelines that follow to review your role in caring for a patient with a head injury.

- Check patient's airway, respirations, pulse rate, and level of consciousness.
- Carefully examine patient for other injuries, such as fractures, lacerations, and abrasions. Pay particular attention to his scalp.
- Immobilize patient's head and neck with a cervical collar, backboard, or sandbags. *Remember:* Don't move him until he's properly immobilized.
- Dress any open wounds.
- Call for medical assistance and stay with patient until help arrives.

Study the chart that follows to familiarize yourself with the causes and signs and symptoms of common head injuries.

NEUROLOGIC
EMERGENCIES

CEREBRAL CONTUSION
(bruising of the brain)

Two types: Coup-contrecoup and acceleration-deceleration
Causes:
Blow to the head that bruises the brain directly; for example, from being hit with a blunt instrument. Such a blow drives the brain into the opposite side of the skull, causing more bruising (coup-contrecoup injury). Or a person's head may be jolted forward, such as in a car accident, causing the brain to slap against the back of the skull. Then, the head stops abruptly, causing the brain to slap against the front of the skull (acceleration-deceleration injury).

Signs and symptoms:
- Variable respirations; may range from normal to ataxic, periodic, or rapid
- Rapid pulse
- Drowsiness
- Disorientation and confusion
- Possibly agitation or violent behavior
- Deteriorating level of or loss of consciousness
- Usually small, equal, and reactive pupils
- Loss of normal eye movement
- Hemiplegia or, if injury's severe, quadriplegia
- Fever, accompanied by diaphoresis
- Possibly severe scalp wounds
- Decerebrate or decorticate posturing

Continued

Guide to Head Injuries
Continued

SKULL FRACTURE

Cause:
Blow to the head, possibly resulting from a fight, fall, or motor vehicle accident

Signs and symptoms:
• Scalp wounds, abrasions, contusions, lacerations, or avulsions. *Note:* Linear fractures may be insidious and require X-ray confirmation.
• Profuse bleeding, especially with an open fracture
• Persistent, localized headaches
• Changes in respiratory patterns; possibly respiratory distress
• Alterations in level of consciousness; possibly loss of consciousness
• Possibly agitation and irritability (with a depressed fracture)
• If bone fragments pierce the dura mater or cerebral cortex, possibly subdural, epidural, or intracerebral hemorrhage or hematoma
• With intracranial or intracerebral hemorrhage, hemiparesis, dizziness, convulsions, projectile vomiting, and decreased pulse rate
• With cranial vault fracture, soft-tissue edema in area of fracture
• With basilar fracture, hemorrhaging from the nose, pharynx, or ears; cerebrospinal fluid drainage from the nose or ears; periorbital ecchymosis without a history of eye trauma; supramastoid ecchymosis (Battle's sign); and sometimes bleeding behind the tympanic membrane (hemotatympanum)
• With sphenoidal fracture, optic nerve damage, possibly resulting in blindness
• With temporal fracture, possibly unilateral deafness or facial paralysis

CONCUSSION (functional impairment of the brain)

Cause:
Blow to the head or face; for example, from a fall, punch, or motor vehicle accident

Signs and symptoms:
• Headache

Continued

NEUROLOGIC
EMERGENCIES

Guide to Head Injuries
Continued

CONCUSSION
Continued

- Dilated pupils
- Restlessness or combativeness
- Drowsiness
- Vertigo
- Nausea
- Weak pulse
- Unusually rapid or slow breathing
- Brief unconsciousness
- Possibly transient amnesia
- Disorientation
- Blurred or double vision (diplopia)

PENETRATING SKULL INJURY (foreign object in the brain)

Cause:
An object, such as a bullet, passing through the skull and lodging in the brain
Signs and symptoms:
- Headache
- Bleeding
- Open wound with protruding object
- Irritability

- Restlessness
- Loss of normal eye movement
- Loss of consciousness

LACERATION
(penetration of skull and brain by an object)

Causes:
Blow to the head, such as from a baseball bat, that may fracture the skull and cause bone fragment to tear brain tissue; in other cases, an object, such as a bullet, passing through the skull and brain but not lodging there
Signs and symptoms:
- Visible open wound at entrance and exit sites
- Loss of consciousness
- Bleeding

FACIAL FRACTURES

Causes:
Direct blow to one of the facial bones, such as the nasal, mandible, maxillae, or zygomatic, usually from trauma, such as from a fall, motor vehicle accident, or contact sport

Continued

NEUROLOGIC EMERGENCIES

Guide to Head Injuries
Continued

FACIAL FRACTURES
Continued

Signs and symptoms:
- Epistaxis, ranging from trickling to full nasal hemorrhage
- Ecchymoses at the affected site

- Soft-tissue edema
- Head and neck pain
- Facial asymmetry from fracture or soft-tissue edema
- Malfunctioning or loss of function of the affected area
- Possibly blood or cerebrospinal fluid drainage from the nose and ears.

Assessing and Intervening for a Spinal Fluid Leak

If you notice fluid leaking from the nose, ear, or mouth, test it with Clinistix. Spinal fluid tests positive for sugar; mucus does not. If blood is tinged, test it for the "halo" sign. On bed linen, spinal fluid usually shows up as a slightly blood-tinged center spot surrounded by a lighter-colored ring. Anytime you're in doubt, put aside stained linen so the doctor can examine it.

Your nursing intervention for a spinal fluid leak should include the following guidelines:
- Keep the patient on absolute bed rest in the correct position. Instruct him not to change his position in any way.
- Is his nose running? Show him how to wipe it with a 4" × 4" gauze pad. Instruct him not to blow it or pick at it.
- Is his ear draining? Cover it lightly with a sterile gauze pad, changing it periodically to examine it for drainage. Do not put any packing inside the ear.

Traumatic Spinal Injuries: General Clinical Considerations

Your patient has suffered a traumatic injury to his vertebral column. Take every precaution to ensure that his injury doesn't become worse and involve the spinal cord. To provide him with proper health care, perform these basic steps:

• Ensure a patent airway. Intubate and suction, as necessary.
• Keep an emergency tracheotomy tray near the patient's bedside.
• Keep the patient in a supine position. Don't allow him to sit up.
• To prevent movement of the patient's spine when transporting, place him on a fracture board. Support the patient's head and neck at all times. Maintain firm, manual, longitudinal head traction during movement. Logroll him to ensure spinal alignment.
• Prevent head rotation by placing sandbags on both sides of the patient's head.

• Assess your patient for additional injuries.
• Watch for signs of shock. If hypotension develops, correct this condition by elevating the patient's legs and starting an I.V., as ordered. Carefully monitor the I.V. flow rate. (If patient's in spinal shock, fluid overload could be dangerous.)
• Perform neurochecks, as directed or as needed.
• Observe for signs of spinal-shock syndrome (the total—but temporary—loss of sensory, motor, autonomic, and reflex activity *below* the level of the spinal cord injury). These signs include: complete flaccid paralysis of all muscles; absence of all spinal reflexes; absence of all cutaneous sensation; absence of all proprioceptive sensation; and transient urinary and fecal retention. If you observe any of these signs, notify the doctor immediately.
• Provide emotional support to the patient and his family.

Guide to Spinal Cord Emergencies

SPINAL CORD TRAUMA

Causes:
• Penetrating injury
• Flexion or extension from fall, diving, or car accident
• In newborn infant, may be caused by traumatic (usually breech) delivery

Signs and symptoms:
• Complete cord transection, resulting in permanent sensory or motor loss below injury level
• Incomplete transection, resulting in variable sensory and motor loss below injury level
• Spinal shock: rapidly decreasing blood pressure, decreased urinary output, and gastric distention

Emergency nursing considerations:
• Immobilize patient immediately (see p. 112).
• Make sure the patient has an open airway, and be prepared to intubate him, if necessary.
• Control any external hemorrhaging.
• Prepare to transfer patient to CircOlectric bed, Stryker frame, or Rotorest frame, as ordered.
• If spinal shock occurs, start I.V. therapy with appropriate solution. Insert Foley catheter to relieve or prevent bladder distention. Insert nasogastric tube to relieve or prevent gastric distention.
• Do not give morphine, because it will depress respirations.

RUPTURED INTRAVERTEBRAL DISC

Cause:
• Trauma

Signs and symptoms:
• When trauma occurs in lumbar area, patient has pain in lower back, radiating down back of one leg. Also, patient's paravertebral muscles are spastic, and his affected leg can't be straightened when his thigh is flexed.
• When trauma occurs in cervical area, patient has neck stiffness and local pain radiating down one arm to fingers.

Emergency nursing considerations:
• Place patient in pelvic or cervical traction, if ordered.
• Prepare patient for myelogram, as ordered.
• Prepare patient for a laminectomy, if ordered.
• Give pain medication, as ordered.

Immobilization and Transfer Techniques

Does your patient have a possible cervical injury? Don't move him until you've immobilized his neck. To maintain immobilization while waiting for help to arrive with a cervical collar, gently grasp your patient's head, taking care to maintain his airway. Now, without applying pressure, cup your hands over his ears. Place your fingers under his jaw, pointing toward each other. Then, using gentle traction, support your patient's head. Now the patient can be placed on a spine board.

Once the spinal cord-injured patient's been admitted to the hospital, move him as little as possible. However, if you must transfer him to a bed or stretcher, follow these guidelines:

Enlist the help of at least four people to transfer your patient. Three should stand on the same side. The leader, preferably a doctor, stands at the patient's head to direct the transfer. When he says "lift," everyone must keep in line and lift together, taking care to maintain the patient's spinal alignment. Once's he's lifted, a fifth person standing at the patient's feet moves the stretcher safely out of the way. During this transfer, the leader may apply manual traction to the patient's head and neck, as described above.

Using Traction to Immobilize a Spinal Cord-Injured Patient

Your spinal cord-injured patient will have to be immobilized for as long as 1 to 3 months. For this, his doctor may use skull tongs, such as Gardner-Wells or Vinke, or halo-vest traction.
• SKULL TONGS immobilize the patient's cervical spine after fracture or dislocation, invasion by tumor or infection, or surgery
• HALO-VEST TRACTION immobilizes the patient's head and neck after cervical spine injury (allows greater mobility than skull tongs; carries less risk of infection)

Spinal Shock

Immediately after spinal cord trauma, expect the patient to undergo a period of spinal shock, or *areflexia,* which is a sudden neurovascular shutdown response. Spinal shock can last from minutes to days, and in some cases as long as several weeks. During this period, watch closely for these problems:

• **Hypotension,** resulting from loss of vascular tone below injury level. You can distinguish it from hypovolemic shock by its associated bradycardia, rather than tachycardia.

• **Hypothermia or hyperthermia,** with no sweating below the injury level. Patient's temperature will be ambient.

• **Flaccid paralysis** below the injury level with bowel and bladder atony. Expect sacral reflexes and priapism, but only in patients with upper motor neuron lesions.

Note: In patients with upper motor neuron lesions, the end of shock is marked by the return of reflexes and by spasticity. Obviously, no reflex activity will return in patients with lower motor neuron lesions.

NEUROLOGIC
EMERGENCIES

Danger Signals in Patients with Spinal Cord Injuries

Any of these conditions in patients with spinal cord injuries may indicate a serious, perhaps life-threatening, situation:

• Increased loss of sensation

• Increased loss of motor functioning

• Severely pounding headache associated with hypertension

• Changes in patterns of respiration.

Taking Seizure Precautions

Whenever you care for a patient with a head injury, you can minimize seizure risk by taking the following precautions:

• Administer anticonvulsant medications on time. Do not omit or increase medication.

• Be sure to use a rectal thermometer, not an oral one, on the seizure-prone patient.

• Pad side rails and headboard to protect him from injury.

• Keep the padded, long side rails in place if he has frequent or generalized seizures, or if he has severe muscle contractions.

• When a patient has an oral endotracheal tube in place, insert an airway to prevent the patient from occluding or biting the endotracheal tube during seizure activity, and to allow for suctioning.

• Keep suction equipment handy in case the patient's airway becomes clogged with oral secretions.

• Monitor the patient's cardiovascular and respiratory status closely to detect hypoxia, which may lead to increased seizure activity.

• Provide emotional support to the patient and family.

• Accompany the seizure-prone patient when he takes a walk.

NEUROLOGIC
EMERGENCIES

Seizure Care

Dealing with a seizure effectively involves both calm observation and quick action. Doing both tasks well is a challenge, but simply knowing *what* to do beforehand helps. When your patient has a seizure, take these actions:

• Stay with the patient and call for assistance.
• Lay the patient flat on the bed or floor. (Don't try to lift a patient onto a bed while he's having a seizure.) Then, try to turn him on his side.
• Loosen tight clothing; for example, his collar and belt.
• Move objects out of the way to protect his head and limbs from injury.
• Guide his movements, if possible, but don't restrain him.
• Don't force open clenched teeth.
• Provide privacy, if possible.

After your patient's seizure, take these actions:

• Place him in bed, if he isn't already.
• Ensure a patent airway by turning him on his side to permit oral drainage. Check his level of consciousness. If it's depressed, insert an oral airway. Suction, as needed.
• If this is the patient's first seizure, notify the doctor immediately. If the patient has had seizures before, notify the doctor immediately only if the seizure activity is prolonged or the patient fails to regain consciousness.
• Check the patient for injury.
• Reorient and reassure the patient as necessary.
• Document everything in your nurses' notes.

Documenting a Seizure

Immediately after your patient's seizure, record the answers to these questions:
- *Onset:* Was it sudden, or preceded by an aura? If preceded by an aura, have the patient describe what he experienced.
- *Duration:* What time did the seizure begin and end?
- *Frequency and number:* Did he have one seizure or several?
- *State of consciousness:* Was the patient unconscious? If so, for how long? Could you arouse him? Note any changes in consciousness.
- *Motor activity:* Where did the motor activity begin? What parts of his body were involved? Was there a pattern of progression to the activity? Describe his movements.
- *Eyes and tongue:* Did they deviate to one side? Did his pupils change in size, shape, equality, or in their reaction to light?
- *Teeth:* Were they clenched or open?
- *Respirations:* What was his respiratory rate and quality? Was he cyanotic?
- *Body activities:* Did he have incontinence, vomiting, salivation, or oral bleeding?
- *Drug response:* If any drugs were administered during the seizure, how did the patient respond? Did the seizure cease? Did it worsen?
- *Seizure awareness:* Is the patient aware of what happened? Did he immediately go into a deep sleep following the seizure? Was he upset? Did he seem ashamed?

Danger Signals

Any of these conditions in patients with seizure disorders may indicate a serious, perhaps life-threatening, situation:
- Severe injury
- Prolonged apnea; cyanosis
- Cardiac dysrhythmias

Initial Burn Assessment Checklist
Assess the ABCs first and intervene appropriately.

CHECK FOR:

• stridor, coughing, hoarseness, sooty sputum, and singed nasal hairs, indicating inhalation injury

• decreased blood pressure and increased pulse rate, indicating impending shock

• diminished peripheral pulses, indicating impaired circulation from edema or thrombosis

• fractures, hemorrhage, or other injuries from a fall or tetanic contractions.

INTERVENE BY:

• dousing the burn with normal saline solution or water, if the burning process hasn't been stopped

• administering supplemental oxygen by face mask

• starting at least two large-bore I.V.s and rapidly infusing fluids

• elevating edematous area

• covering the patient with a sheet or blanket to prevent hypothermia

• inserting an indwelling (Foley) catheter and a nasogastric tube.

PREPARE FOR:

• intubation and mechanical ventilation

• cutdown with central I.V. line insertion

• cleansing and debridement

• bedside X-rays.

TRAUMATIC
EMERGENCIES

Calculating Extent of the Burn

	Ante-rior	Poste-rior
head	_____	_____
neck	_____	_____
right arm	_____	_____
rt. forearm	_____	_____
right hand	_____	_____
left arm	_____	_____
lt. forearm	_____	_____
left hand	_____	_____
trunk	_____	_____
buttock	_____	_____
perineum	_____	_____
right thigh	_____	_____
right leg	_____	_____
right foot	_____	_____
left thigh	_____	_____
left leg	_____	_____
left foot	_____	_____
Subtotal	_____	_____
% Total area burned		_____

To calculate the extent of a patient's burn, follow these steps:
1) Shade the body diagrams on the opposite page so they reflect the burn on each part of the patient's body, front and back. If only a portion of a body section is burned, shade only a portion of that area.
2) The numbers on the diagrams represent the percentage of the body that's burned. Record the numbers of the area you shade in the table at right. If only a fraction of an area is burned, divide the number by that fraction, and record *that* number in the chart.

Remember that as children grow up, the proportions of their bodies change. These changes occur primarily in the head, thighs, and legs, so the percentage of the body these areas represent varies according to age. Use the age table on the opposite page to calculate the correct percentage for these areas.
3) Consider all parts of the body and then add the numbers to obtain a subtotal for anterior and posterior burns. Add these figures for the percentage of total body area burned.
4) When you gauge a burn's severity, consider the depth as well as the size.

Continued

Calculating Extent of the Burn
Continued

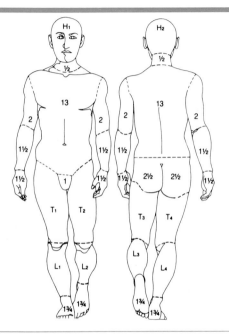

PATIENT'S AGE	0	1	5	10	15	Adult
H (1 or 2) = ½ of the head	9½	8½	6½	5½	4½	3½
T (1, 2, 3 or 4) = ½ of a thigh	2¾	3¼	4	4¼	4½	4¾
L (1, 2, 3 or 4) = ½ of a leg	2½	2½	2¾	3	3¼	3½

Guidelines for Fluid Replacement

While fluids are being replaced, assess your patient's response and use it to titrate the rate of fluid replacement. But use caution in giving massive fluid replacement to elderly and pediatric patients and to anyone with a history of heart failure. Osmotic diuretics or low-dose dopamine infusion may be necessary to maintain adequate urine output and to prevent fluid overload in these patients, or to aid myoglobin clearance in patients with deep-muscle damage.

ASSESSMENT FACTORS	NURSING CONSIDERATIONS
Intake and output (hourly)	Maintain minimum urine output at 30 to 50 ml/hr in an adult, 0.5 to 1 ml/kg/hr in a child, or 70 to 100 ml/hr in a patient with a deep-burn injury affecting muscle tissue, to prevent renal failure from myoglobinuria.
Vital signs (every 15 minutes to hourly)	Maintain the patient's blood pressure above 90/60. Increase the fluid infusion rate and notify the doctor if the patient's blood pressure drops more than 20 mm Hg below baseline or if his pulse rises above 110 beats/minute.
Mental status (continuously)	Note changes such as restlessness, confusion, or agitation in a previously quiet patient, indicating poor cerebral perfusion.
Body weight (same time daily)	Expect the patient to gain weight during the first 48 to 72 hours, due to third-space fluid shifting. Thereafter, expect the patient's weight to slowly decrease toward normal dry weight.

Continued

TRAUMATIC
EMERGENCIES

Guidelines for Fluid Replacement
Continued

ASSESSMENT FACTORS	NURSING CONSIDERATIONS
Respiratory status (hourly)	Check the patient's breath sounds for rales, and note dyspnea, which may indicate fluid overload. If rales or dyspnea is present, decrease the fluid administration rate and notify the doctor.
Cardiac status (frequently)	Monitor the EKG continuously with an elderly patient or a patient with a history of heart failure, and auscultate heart sounds at least hourly; notify the doctor if rales, dysrhythmias, or abnormal heart sounds—which may indicate fluid overload—develop.
Blood tests (at least daily) • hematocrit • sodium	Notify the doctor if the patient's values are elevated (possibly indicating underhydration) or decreased (possibly indicating overhydration). He may change the infusion rate and the type of fluid administered and may order a blood transfusion. (Note: Expect an initial rise in hematocrit values.)
Urine specific gravity (every 4 hours)	If elevated, expect to increase the infusion rate; or if decreased, to decrease the infusion rate.

Continued

TRAUMATIC EMERGENCIES

Guidelines for Fluid Replacement
Continued

Your patient with serious burns needs massive fluid replacement—especially for the first several days postburn. Expect to give a combination of crystalloids (such as dextrose in water) or colloids to meet your patient's fluid needs. Your hospital may use one of the following formulas to calculate your patient's initial fluid requirements, depending on his age, his ability to tolerate fluids, and the preferred formula.

FORMULA	ELECTROLYTE-CONTAINING SOLUTION	COLLOIDS	DEXTROSE
FIRST 24 HOURS POSTBURN			
Baxter (Parkland)	Ringer's lactate— 4 ml/kg/% burn	Not used	Not used
Hypertonic sodium solution	Volume of fluid containing 250 mEq of sodium per liter to maintain hourly urinary output of 30 ml	Not used	Not used
Modified Brooke	Ringer's lactate— 2 ml/kg/% burn	Not used	Not used
Burn budget of F.D. Moore	Ringer's lactate— 1,000 to 4,000 ml; 0.5 normal saline— 1,200 ml	7.5% of body weight	1,500 to 5,000 ml
Evans	Normal saline— 1 ml/kg/% burn	1 ml/kg/% burn	2,000 ml
Brooke	Ringer's lactate— 1.5 ml/kg/% burn	0.5 ml/kg/% burn	2,000 ml

Continued

TRAUMATIC EMERGENCIES

Guidelines for Fluid Replacement
Continued

FORMULA	ELECTROLYTE-CONTAINING SOLUTION	COLLOIDS	DEXTROSE
SECOND 24 HOURS POSTBURN			
Burn budget of F.D. Moore	Ringer's lactate—1,000 to 4,000 ml; 0.5 normal saline—1,200 ml	2.5% of body weight	1,500 to 5,000 ml
Evans	½ of first 24-hour requirement	½ of first 24-hour requirement	2,000 ml
Brooke	½ to ¾ of first 24-hour requirement	½ to ¾ of first 24-hour requirement	2,000 ml
Parkland	Not used	20% to 60% of calculated plasma volume (within 24 to 32 hours)	As necessary to maintain urinary output
Hypertonic sodium solution	⅓ isotonic salt solution orally, up to 3,500-ml limit	Not used	Not used
Modified Brooke	Not used	0.3 to 0.5 ml/kg/% burn	As necessary to maintain urinary output

Avoiding Dextrose in Early Fluid Replacement

Don't give dextrose to your burn patient during the first 24 hours of fluid replacement. Why? Because dextrose isn't effective as the primary fluid replacement for this patient. It doesn't remain in the vascular space, where fluid's needed—instead, it passes into the interstitial space. What's more, your patient can't metabolize the dextrose given in massive fluid replacement; he's already overloaded with internal glucose released during his stress response to the burn, and the effectiveness of his insulin is decreased. An isotonic-balanced electrolyte solution, such as Ringer's lactate, is preferred, since it has an electrolyte balance similar to that of blood.

All About Temporary Skin Grafts

A patient with deep partial-thickness or full-thickness burns needs skin grafts to prevent infection and to promote healing of the wounds. These grafts may be applied as soon as eschar is removed.

Types of temporary grafts include:
• allografts (homografts), consisting of human skin from a cadaver (usually obtained from a skin bank)
• xenografts (heterografts), consisting of animal skin (commonly pigskin)
• biosynthetic grafts, consisting of a combination of collagen and synthetics.

Special Consideration

As a nurse, you know that patients with burns receive virtually all their medications I.V. Why? Because in these patients, widespread shifts in body fluids make absorption by the subcutaneous and I.M. routes erratic.

But one exception exists. It's tetanus toxoid, which is always given I.M. to burn patients—in fact, to *all* patients. So don't be surprised when your burn patient's medication order reads: "Tetanus toxoid I.M." It's the exception to the "I.V.-only" rule.

TRAUMATIC
EMERGENCIES

How to Care for Chemical Burns

In most cases, chemical burns result from home or industrial accidents. Tissue damage is usually caused by direct chemical action and its subsequent release of heat energy. The burn's severity depends on the chemical's concentration and the length of time it remains on the victim's skin. No wonder, then, that your prompt, effective action is so important if you're at the scene of the accident. Here's what to do:

First, immediately dilute the chemical by flushing the burned area with copious amounts of water or normal saline solution. Then, remove any clothing surrounding the burned area. This will prevent further tissue damage from chemicals that remain in your patient's garments.

Find out which chemical or combination of chemicals caused his burn. Make sure this information is documented so other health-care professionals can begin specific treatment when your patient arrives in the emergency department. Check the patient for any other injuries and document these also. Continue flushing the burn until you transport him to the ED, or until he's no longer in your care.

Important: Never flush a phosphorous burn with water or any type of solution. Doing so could cause tissue sloughing. Instead, gently soak the affected area with water.

Nursing Tip

If your burned patient's peripheral edema or severe hypotension prevents you from palpating his peripheral pulses or auscultating his blood pressure with a stethoscope, try using a Doppler ultrasonic flowmeter. Here's what to do:

Apply coupling gel to the Doppler's probe. Tilt the probe at a 45° angle to your patient's skin, then slowly move it in a circular motion until you hear an optimal arterial or venous flow sound. Count the sounds for 60 seconds to determine your patient's pulse rate. Next, apply a blood pressure cuff and inflate it until the arterial sound disappears. Then slowly deflate the cuff until the sound reappears, and note the systolic pressure reading on the sphygmomanometer.

TRAUMATIC
EMERGENCIES

How to Care for Radiation Burns

Caring for a radiation burn victim? You'll have to make special provisions before and after he arrives. Why? Because radioactive contamination, usually present in such a burn, creates a serious health hazard for all who come in contact with the victim. *Remember:* Radioactive decontamination guidelines differ, so always follow your state's and hospital's policies. Also keep in mind that this information *does not apply* to patients suffering skin irritation from radiation therapy.

Here's how to prepare for the victim's arrival:
• Prepare an isolated area in which to treat him. Make sure there's enough room for health-care professionals, disposal hampers, and the stretcher. Enclose the area with lead-lined shields. If that's impossible, make arrangements to care for the patient in your hospital's X-ray department. Next, cover the floor of the area with newspapers or other absorbent paper. Tape the paper in place with masking tape.
• Notify hospital maintenance personnel that you may want to shut off the air-circulating system in the area.
• Make sure you and the other team members are wearing surgical caps, masks, gowns, gloves, and booties.

After the victim arrives, follow these steps:
• Use a Geiger counter to check his contamination level while he's still on the ambulance stretcher. Then, get him to the shielded area immediately.
• When he's inside the area, do a quick head-to-toe assessment. Treat any life-threatening injuries and administer tetanus toxoid, as ordered.
• Save any clothes you remove from the patient, as well as the bedding from the ambulance. Also, save any metal objects the patient is wearing, such as jewelry, a belt buckle, or dental appliances. Instruct another health-care professional to label

Continued

TRAUMATIC EMERGENCIES

How to Care for Radiation Burns
Continued

each item with the patient's name, his location within the hospital, the date, and the time. Retain each item in an individual lead or plastic container that's been clearly marked RADIO-ACTIVE: DO NOT DISCARD.

• If you suspect the patient may have inhaled or ingested radioactive materials, save any blood, urine, or vomitus. Place it in an individual container and label as explained above.

• Cleanse radiation burns with soap and water. If the patient's entire body is contaminated, shower him in a lead-lined shower. When you cleanse your patient, pay special attention to hairy body surfaces, orifices, and skin folds.

• To decontaminate your patient, you'll probably have to wash or shower him several times. Measure and record his contamination level each time. Continue until the contamination level registers zero on the Geiger counter.

• Transfer the radiation burn patient to the proper unit, where his burns will be treated like thermal burns. After that, you'll have to decontaminate yourself and anyone else who's been in contact with him. To do this, follow the steps above.

Splinting Technique

Splint palmar burns so that the fingers extend and the thumb abducts. To pad and protect the hand, first apply one layer of a fine-mesh gauze and one layer of Kerlix around palm and fingers. Then anchor the splint at the wrist so that the metacarpophalangeal joints extend one inch beyond the bend in the splint. Wrap Kerlix around the entire hand to secure the splint in place.

Documenting Emergency Burn Care Properly

To document the care you give a burn patient in the ED, you must collect as much information as you can about the accident, the patient's past medical history, and his present physical condition. Use a data collection sheet and fill in every blank. Make sure you find out answers to the following questions:

• How did the burn occur? What kind of care was given to the patient before he arrived at the hospital?

• Has he been taking any medication?

• Does he have any chronic illnesses or allergies?

Record the baseline data you'll get from various diagnostic tests. Take time to record specific information accurately. The health-care professionals who care for him later will need all the information you can provide. Then, make sure the properly filled out data collection sheet accompanies him when he's transferred.

Encouraging Your Patient's Cooperation

When your patient with serious burns realizes the difficult, painful, and frustrating obstacles he faces during treatment and rehabilitation, he'll probably feel completely overwhelmed. Unfortunately, his despair may translate into refusal to cooperate in his treatment.

To encourage his cooperation, try establishing a contract with him each time you begin a difficult procedure.

Why a contract? Because, if your patient has a part in planning his care, he'll begin regaining some sense of control over his life. And, besides reminding him of his responsibility for keeping up his end of the agreement,

a contract lets the patient know he can count on *you* to maintain *your* part of the agreement. A contract also gives both of you a chance to recognize each milestone of his progress and to feel a sense of accomplishment when difficult procedures are finished. Of course, day-to-day, informal, verbal contracts will do. Here are some guidelines:

• First, identify a short-term achievable goal.

• Next, explain to the patient why the goal is important.

• Then explain what you expect from your patient.

• Finally, be sure to explain what your patient can expect from *you.*

Initial Shock Assessment Checklist

Assess the ABCs first and intervene appropriately.

CHECK FOR:

• altered mental status, indicating decreased cerebral tissue perfusion (early sign)

• tachycardia, indicating decreased cardiac output (early sign)

• tachypnea, indicating poor tissue perfusion (early sign) and acidosis (late sign)

• pale, cool, and clammy skin, indicating compensatory sympathetic response (early sign); or warm, flushed, dry skin, indicating vasodilation (early sign of septic shock).

INTERVENE BY:

• positioning the patient properly

• administering supplemental oxygen

• inserting at least one large-bore I.V. and administering fluids

• taking a 12-lead EKG and establishing cardiac monitoring

• administering appropriate medications, such as antibiotics, vasoactive drugs, or corticosteroids.

PREPARE FOR:

• blood transfusion, if the patient's hemorrhaging

• central venous pressure line insertion

• Swan-Ganz catheter and arterial line insertion

• medical antishock trousers (MAST suit) application

• autotransfusion

• colloid and crystalloid replacement.

TRAUMATIC
EMERGENCIES

Combating Shock: Some Guidelines

Do you know how to act on the signs and symptoms shown on page 129? The chart below will give you specific instructions. Study it carefully. In addition, remember these guidelines that apply to all types of shock:

• Call the doctor immediately.
• Check to be sure the patient has an open airway and adequate circulation. Start cardiopulmonary resuscitation (CPR), if necessary.
• Correct the cause of shock.
• Remain with the patient. Provide a calm, quiet atmosphere, if possible, and give emotional support.
• Record blood pressure, pulse rate, and other vital signs at least once every 15 minutes.
• Keep the patient covered with a light blanket.
• Begin I.V. therapy, as ordered.
• Draw venous blood for type and cross match, complete blood count (CBC), and serum electrolytes, as ordered.
• Obtain arterial blood for arterial blood gas measurements. Treat any acid-base disturbances that may occur, as ordered.
• Assist doctor with insertion of central venous pressure (CVP) line for CVP readings and fluid replacement.
• Monitor intake and output. Insert an indwelling (Foley) catheter to measure urinary output, if ordered. If output is less than 30 ml/hour, carefully increase fluid infusion, as ordered, but be alert for signs of overhydration.

HYPOVOLEMIC SHOCK

Possible causes:
Decreased blood volume resulting from blood loss, severe dehydration, third space sequestration (as in burns or pancreatitis), or abnormal fluid loss (for example, excessive vomiting or diarrhea)

Nursing interventions:
• Place patient in a supine position and elevate his feet 20° to 30°.
• Administer low-percentage oxygen.
• To increase circulating blood volume, increase I.V. fluid rate until blood or blood products are available. Give volume expanders, such as albumin, if ordered.

Continued

Combating Shock: Some Guidelines
Continued

CARDIOGENIC SHOCK

Possible causes:
Myocardial infarction, pericardial tamponade, cardiac arrest, or pulmonary artery embolism, resulting from stress of surgery and/or anesthesia

Nursing interventions:
• Administer oxygen.
• To improve cardiac output, administer an inotropic drug such as dopamine hydrochloride (Intropin*), I.V. drip, as ordered.
• Place the patient on cardiac monitor, or obtain an immediate electrocardiogram (EKG).
• Prepare the patient for transfer to the intensive care unit (ICU). Prepare him emotionally for procedures he may undergo in the ICU; for example, pulmonary artery catheter insertion or intra-aortic balloon pump insertion.

SEPTIC SHOCK

Septic shock may produce these additional signs and symptoms: low-grade fever (except in burn patients who may be hypothermic), nausea, vomiting, abdominal cramps or distention, elevated white blood cell count, and increased blood urea nitrogen (BUN).

Possible causes:
Cell destruction from endotoxins caused by a bacterial infection (usually gram-negative)

Nursing interventions:
• Administer oxygen.
• Establish I.V. line.
• Obtain specimens for culture and sensitivity tests, as ordered.
• Administer a broad-spectrum antibiotic, as ordered.
• If ordered, give patient a steroid, such as dexamethasone (Decadron*), to reduce inflammation and improve cardiovascular function.
• Be prepared to transfer the patient to the ICU.

NEUROGENIC SHOCK

Possible causes:
Abnormal blood vessel dilation from cervical fracture, concussion, spinal cord injury, or spinal anesthetic

Nursing interventions:
• Keep patient supine. If you suspect cerebral edema, reposition him in a 20° to 30° Fowler position.
• Perform frequent neurochecks.
• Administer large volumes of fluid to correct hypovolemia.

TRAUMATIC EMERGENCIES

*Available in both the United States and in Canada

Dealing with Hypovolemic Shock

Any patient who loses a large amount of body fluid runs the risk of developing hypovolemic shock. To reverse this potentially lethal complication, you must give prompt, effective emergency care, as detailed in the chart below.

SIGNS AND SYMPTOMS

- Cold, clammy, or pale skin
- Low blood pressure
- Decreased temperature
- Increased pulse
- Increased respiration rate
- Blood and fluid loss exceeds 20% of total circulatory volume
- Restlessness

PHYSIOLOGIC CHANGES

- Vasoconstriction, reducing blood flow to vital organs
- Inadequate oxygenation of individual cells (tissue perfusion)
- Increased lactic acid
- Impaired renal and hepatic function
- Metabolic acidosis

WHAT TO DO

- Unless you suspect head injury, place the patient in a supine position. Elevate the patient's legs 20° to 30° provided, of course, he has no leg injuries.

- Check for an open airway and adequate circulation. Start CPR, if necessary.
- Give low-pressure (24%) oxygen by face mask or nasal airway to ensure adequate tissue perfusion.
- Keep patient covered with a light blanket.
- Insert a Foley catheter to measure urine output. If output's less than 30 ml/hr, increase flow rate of I.V., but watch for signs of overhydration.
- Draw arterial blood sample to measure blood gas levels. Have venous blood drawn for complete blood count (CBC), electrolytes, type, and cross match.
- Record vital signs every 15 minutes.
- Using large-bore catheters, start I.V.s in both arms or legs. *Caution:* Has the patient suffered abdominal trauma? Don't use his legs for infusion sites. If you do, the fluid may escape through ruptured vessels into his abdomen.
- Assist the doctor with insertion of a central line for CVP reading and fluid replacement.

Caring for Specific Problems: Some Tips

Sometimes a patient who's hemorrhaging severely has problems that require special attention. For example:

If he's on anticoagulant or aspirin therapy:
• Give the appropriate antidote, as prescribed by the doctor. To neutralize 75 to 90 units of heparin, give 1 mg protamine sulfate*, diluted 1%, I.V. push over 1 to 3 minutes. To neutralize warfarin sodium (Coumadin*), give 2.5 to 10 mg vitamin K$_1$* (phytonadione) I.M., subcutaneously, or I.V. push not to exceed 1 mg per minute.

If he's bleeding from a major abdominal vessel:
• Don't administer I.V. fluid in either leg because the infusing I.V. fluid may escape from the damaged vessel into abdominal or retroperitoneal space.

If his neck is injured:
• Give I.V. fluids in the arm that's on the opposite side of the neck injury to keep the infusing I.V. fluid from leaving the damaged vessel and entering the intracranial or the thoracic space.

If he's hemorrhaging from a fractured arm or leg:
• Apply a plastic air splint.
• Avoid raising the fractured limb.

If he has hemophilia:
• Depending on the doctor's orders, administer one or all of the following: plasma, vitamin K$_1$, or antihemophilic factor (AHF), 10 to 20 units/ kg, I.V. push or infusion every 8 to 24 hours.
• Never give aspirin, or any drug containing aspirin, for pain.
• Use a finger stick to draw blood for coagulation studies.
• If your patient refuses needed blood or blood products because of personal or religious beliefs, consider giving a plasma expander, like dextran I.V., per doctor's order. If the patient's a minor, the doctor may request a court order for permission to perform the appropriate lifesaving treatment.

If your patient develops disseminated intravascular coagulation:
• Observe him closely for occult bleeding.
• Give plasma, platelets, or packed red blood cells, per doctor's order.
• If a blood transfusion proves ineffective, give anticoagulant therapy I.V., per doctor's order. However, before giving an anticoagulant, check the patient's blood coagulation studies for baseline information. Expect the prothrombin time (PT) and the partial thromboplastin time (PTT) to be prolonged in the late stages of DIC.

*Available in the United States and in Canada.

TRAUMATIC EMERGENCIES

How to Control a Hemorrhage

• For a wound of the scalp or temple, compress the temporal artery.
• For a wound of the lower face (below the eyes), apply pressure to the facial artery along the lower border of the mandible.
• For a neck wound, compress the wound site. Do not compress the carotid artery, as this could cause stroke.
• For a shoulder wound or hemorrhage of the upper arm, compress the subclavian artery against the clavicle.
• For a wound of the lower part of the upper arm or of the elbow, press the brachial artery against the humerus.
• For foot wounds, compress the entire network of arteries in the ankle.
• For a wound of the lower arm, press the ulnar and radial arteries at the antecubital fossa.
• For hand wounds, press the ulnar and radial arteries at the wrist.
• For thigh wounds, apply great pressure to the femoral artery against the femur.
• For wounds of the lower leg, apply pressure to the popliteal artery, behind the knee.

Nursing Tip

Finding a vein: As you know, your first priority for a patient in hypovolemic shock is beginning fluid replacement therapy. But when you prepare to do a venipuncture for an I.V., don't be surprised if you can't find a vein. Shock causes your patient's veins to constrict, making them difficult to locate. Here are some tips to help you find a vein when your patient's in shock:
• Drape his arm over the side of his bed so it's below the level of his heart; then apply a soft-rubber tourniquet. This will inhibit venous return and cause the arm veins to fill with blood, bringing them to the surface.
• If you can't locate an arm or hand vein, try to find a vein in your patient's legs or feet.
• If you still can't find a vein, try a blind stick—attempt a venipuncture at a spot where you expect a vein to be, based on your knowledge of vein locations and previous experience.

Do's and Don'ts for Using MAST Effectively

MAST (Medical Anti-Shock Trousers) counteracts bleeding and hypovolemia by slowing or stopping arterial bleeding; by forcing any available
blood from the lower body to the heart, brain, and other vital organs;
and by preventing return of the available circulating blood volume to the
lower extremities.

DO'S

• While patient is wearing MAST,
monitor blood pressure, apical
and radial pulse rates, and respirations; check extremities for pe-
dal pulses, color, warmth, and
numbness; and make sure MAST
is not too constricting.

• Take MAST off only when a
doctor is present, fluids are available for transfusion, and anesthesia and surgical teams are
available.

• To clean, wash with warm soap
and water, air dry, and store.

DON'TS

• Don't apply MAST if positions of
wounds show or suggest major intrathoracic or intracranial vascular
injury; or if patient has open extremity bleeding, pulmonary
edema, or trauma above the level
of MAST application.

• When cleaning, don't autoclave
or clean with solvents.

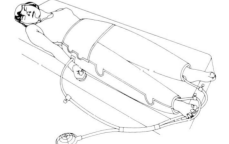

Cardiogenic Shock: Taking the First Steps

Do you suspect that your patient is going into cardiogenic shock? Take these steps:
• Call the doctor immediately.
• Administer oxygen to promote adequate tissue oxygenation.
• Start an I.V. or check the patency of the existing I.V. line.
• Insert an indwelling (Foley) catheter, and measure urine output frequently.
• Draw blood specimens for arterial blood gas measurements and cardiac isoenzyme studies, as ordered.
• Obtain a 12-lead EKG to help locate myocardial damage.
• As ordered, administer I.V. drugs, such as dopamine hydrochloride (a vasoconstrictor that—depending on dosage—may increase cardiac output, blood pressure, and renal blood flow), norepinephrine (if your patient needs a more potent vasoconstrictor), or nitroprusside sodium (a vasodilator that may reduce preload and afterload).
• Place your patient in low Fowler's position. However, if he's unconscious or semiconscious, place him in a supine position to encourage maximum blood flow to the brain.
• Assist with tracheal intubation, if indicated.
• Prepare your patient for transfer to the cardiac care unit (CCU). There, he'll receive continuous cardiac and arterial blood pressure monitoring, intracardiac pressure monitoring with a pulmonary artery catheter, and (if necessary) artificial ventilation.
• Provide emotional support to your patient and his family. In easy-to-understand terms, explain all procedures as well as what to expect after the patient's transfer to the CCU.

What Causes Cardiogenic Shock?

Although left ventricular failure from myocardial infarction is the most common cause of cardiogenic shock, it's not the *only* cause. Other possible causes include:
• Chronic, progressive heart diseases
• Injury or disease causing mechanical failure
• Obstruction of venous return reducing preload
• Dysrhythmias

Neurogenic Shock: Collecting the Facts

Thoroughly assessing a patient with suspected neurogenic shock is an essential and ongoing part of your nursing responsibility. You'll need to observe, evaluate, and document his condition from the moment he enters your care. The details you observe may provide your first clues to possible neurogenic shock. Ask yourself these questions:
• Why was the patient admitted?
• Has he (or could he have) experienced spinal cord trauma?
• Is he experiencing motor or sensory impairment in his arms or legs? Does he complain of numbness, weakness, or a tingling sensation?
• Has he (or could he have) experienced head trauma? If so, what's his level of consciousness? Can he follow simple commands? Does he respond appropriately to questions?
• Did he have surgery? If so, what type of anesthesia did he undergo? General? Spinal?
• If he had a general anesthetic, did he experience *deep* anesthesia?
• Does he have a history of hypoglycemia?
• Is he receiving insulin or an oral antidiabetic drug?

Neurogenic Shock Priorities

Although neurogenic shock is commonly of short duration and self-limiting, it can affect your patient's cardiovascular and respiratory systems profoundly during its course. So your first priority is to support these systems:
• Give your patient supplemental oxygen as needed.
• Keep your patient supine to prevent orthostatic hypotension from the relative hypovolemia his increased vascular capacity may cause.
• Start I.V. fluids, as ordered, to expand your patient's intravascular volume.
• Insert an indwelling catheter, as ordered.

Recognizing Toxic Shock Syndrome

Toxic shock syndrome (TSS) is an acute form of septic shock caused by infection with *Staphylococcus aureus*—a gram-positive bacterium that may invade any part of your patient's body. Once *S. aureus* has invaded every part of your patient's body, the bacteria secrete enterotoxins that cause TSS.

TSS is most common in menstruating women using tampons, but it strikes patients of either sex and any age. On the average, two new cases are reported each day in the United States, and two deaths occur each month.

TSS is difficult to recognize and diagnose. No positive diagnostic test exists, the onset of TSS is insidious, and its systemic signs and symptoms mimic many other diseases, including viral influenza, food poisoning, scarlet fever, Kawasaki disease, and Rocky Mountain spotted fever.

Remember to consider the possibility of TSS whenever you see a patient with this clinical picture:
• fever above 102° F. (38.9° C.)
• systolic blood pressure below 90 mm Hg
• diffuse rash
• signs and symptoms indicating involvement of at least three body areas (mucous membranes or GI, musculoskeletal, renal, hepatic, hematologic, or central nervous systems)
• negative blood and cerebrospinal fluid culture tests; negative serologic tests for measles, leptospirosis, and Rocky Mountain spotted fever
• positive results of testing for *S. aureus* cultured from the nose, throat, vagina, or any wound
• desquamation (especially of the palms and soles) a week or more after the onset of signs and symptoms.

TRAUMATIC
EMERGENCIES

Some Drugs Commonly Used in Shock

ADRENERGICS

Dobutamine hydrochloride (Dobutrex):
250-mg vial diluted and added to 250, 500, or 1,000 ml of dextrose 5% in water. Titrate drip rate to 2.5 to 10 mcg/kg/minute.

Dopamine hydrochloride (Intropin):
200- or 400-mg ampul added to 250 or 500 ml dextrose 5% in water, normal saline solution, combination of dextrose and saline solution, or lactated Ringer's injection. Titrate to 2 to 5 mcg/kg/minute up to 50 mcg/kg/minute.

Norepinephrine injection (Levophed):
Initially 8 to 12 mcg/minute by I.V. infusion. Average maintenance dose 2 to 4 mcg/minute.

Metaraminol bitartrate (Aramine):
0.5 to 5 mg I.V. bolus followed by 15 to 100 mg in 500 ml of normal saline or dextrose 5% in water. Titrate infusion rate to desired blood pressure reading.

DIGITALIS GLYCOSIDES

Digoxin (Lanoxin):
0.5 to 1 mg I.V.

Deslanoside (Cedilanid-D):
1.2 to 1.6 mg I.V. in divided doses over 24 hours

SYSTEMIC BUFFER

Sodium bicarbonate:
7.5% or 8.4% solution, 1 to 3 mEq/kg I.V.

ANTIHISTAMINE

Diphenhydramine (Benadryl):
50 to 100 mg I.V., 50 mg P.O. every 6 hours

SPASMOLYTIC AGENT

Aminophylline:
500 mg in 250 ml dextrose 5% in water (2 mg/2.2 kg of body weight)

CORTICOSTEROIDS

Dexamethasone phosphate (Decadron Phosphate):
1 to 6 mg/kg I.V. single dose or 40 mg I.V. every 2 to 6 hours, as necessary

Hydrocortisone (Solu-Cortef):
500 mg to 2 g every 2 to 6 hours.

TRAUMATIC EMERGENCIES

Precautions for Drugs Used in Shock

Corticosteroids:
- Watch for GI bleeding

Isuprel:
- Monitor EKG with defibrillator at bedside.
- Slow or stop infusion if heart rate exceeds 110 beats/minute.
- Measure urine output and BP every 15 minutes.
- Do not use with epinephrine.

Intropin:
- Monitor EKG for ventricular dysrhythmias.
- Maintain CVP at 10 to 15 cm H_2O.
- Check urine output every 30 minutes.
- Do not add to alkaline solutions.

Digitalis:
- Monitor pulse and EKG constantly.

Vasopressors:
- Monitor EKG for PVCs.
- Watch for ventricular decompensation and pulmonary edema.
- Stop if headache, chest pain, nausea, or hypotension develops.

Heparin:
- Monitor with partial thromboplastin times (PTT).
- Maintain at 2½ times control.

Systemic buffers:
- Give slowly.
- Monitor EKG.

Aminophylline:
- Give slowly.

TRAUMATIC
EMERGENCIES

Special Consideration

Is your patient at risk? Consider *any* patient under physical or emotional stress to be a candidate for shock. Be alert if he:
- has a serious injury or infection
- is vomiting or has diarrhea
- has any form of diabetes
- is very young or elderly
- is experiencing severe pain
- has a bowel obstruction
- is undergoing any procedure that causes rapid decompression of an organ or rapid fluid loss from a body cavity
- has undergone anesthesia.

Initial Musculoskeletal Assessment Checklist

Assess the ABCs first and intervene appropriately.

CHECK FOR:

• deformity, local swelling, decreased range of motion, immobility, or bruises, indicating fracture or dislocation
• poor capillary refill, absent or diminished pulses, pallor or cool skin, possibly indicating vascular compromise
• paralysis, numbness, or decreased sensation, indicating nerve injury.

INTERVENE BY:

• immobilizing the injured part
• preserving an amputated part.

PREPARE FOR:

• compartment pressure measurement
• traction
• surgical interventions
• transfer to a replantation center.

Assessment Questions

Most musculoskeletal injuries result from traumatic events. But remember, for the patient who's elderly or has bone disease, even a minor insult—such as stepping off a curb the wrong way—can cause a major musculoskeletal injury. Be sure to ask your patient what he heard and felt at the time of the injury:

• Did he hear a snapping, crack-ing, grating, or popping sound?
• Can he describe any other sensations he noticed?
• Could he move the affected area right after the injury?
• When and where did the injury occur?
• What steps were taken to manage the injury before he arrived at the hospital?

TRAUMATIC EMERGENCIES

Identifying Fracture Signs and Symptoms

Specific fracture signs and symptoms vary, depending on the fracture type (incomplete, complete, closed, open, non-displaced, displaced, transverse, spiral, linear, comminuted, impacted, compression, avulsion, depression) and its location. Of course, if a patient's bones are protruding from an open, bleeding wound, you'll know he has a fracture. But a *closed* fracture can be much more difficult to assess visually.

Look for these physical signs and symptoms that generally accompany a fracture:

• deformity or shortening of the injured area

• localized discoloration and edema

• pain in injured area (especially at time of injury occurrence)

• patient's tendency to guard the injured area by holding it in a protected position

• tenderness of injured area lasting several hours to several days after the injury occurs

• presence of crepitation (crackling sound) during skin palpation

• decrease or complete loss of muscle power at injured area

• presence of grating sound when testing for range of motion during standard assessment.

If a grating sound is detected, notify the doctor immediately. Avoid moving the limb any further. Doing so can cause additional injury and pain. *Special Note:* Never deliberately test range of motion if you suspect a fracture.

Types of Fractures

Incomplete:
Break extends only partially through the bone; for example, in a greenstick fracture (common in children), bone splinters fibers on one side of the bone, leaving the other side intact

Complete:
Bone breaks into two or more pieces

Closed (simple):
Overlying skin remains unbroken

Open (compound):
Wound is present overlying the fracture, creating the risk of infection

Nondisplaced:
Fractured bones remain in alignment

Displaced:
Break knocks bone ends out of alignment, creating the risk of muscle contractures and deformities

Transverse:
Break runs transversely across the bone shaft

Spiral:
Break winds around bone like a coil

Linear:
Break runs the length of the bone

Comminuted:
Bone shatters or is compressed into fragments

Impacted:
Bone ends are driven into each other

Compression:
Bone collapses (vertebrae) under excessive pressure

Avulsion:
Overexertion tears a muscle or ligament away from a bone, pulling a small bone fragment with it

Depression:
Trauma drives bone fragments inward (usually refers to a skull fracture)

Do's and Don'ts of Fracture Care

• Do ease your patient's pain and distress by explaining what you're going to do.
• Don't straighten a severely angulated extremity before immobilizing it.
• Don't push protruding bone ends into your patient's skin when you immobilize the injured extremity.
• Do remember to pad the splint before you apply it.
• Don't constrict your patient's circulation when you immobilize his injured part.
• Do check your patient's immobilized extremity every 15 minutes for possible temperature and color changes.
• Do elevate the patient's injured extremity above his heart after you splint it, to decrease risk of edema.
• Do look for signs that your patient may have internal hemorrhaging, increasing pain, or shock. For example, stay alert for personality changes, restlessness, or irritability.
• Do give your patient medication for pain, as ordered by the doctor.
• Do notify the doctor if you have problems with your patient's traction device.

Types of Traction

The doctor may order traction for a patient to treat a fracture or dislocation, to decrease muscle spasms, or to immobilize an injury before surgery.

Skin traction is used to treat fractures in small children or to reduce pain in adults by temporarily immobilizing their injuries.

Skeletal traction is used to treat long-bone fractures and cervical spine fractures.

Both types of traction work by exerting a pulling force on a body part. For skin traction, the doctor connects the weight system to a bandage made of moleskin and elastic; for skeletal traction, he connects it to a pin or wire. (You may be asked to apply some forms of skin traction.)

Checking for Fat Embolism

Fat embolism, a potentially fatal complication of arm or leg fractures, may follow the release of fat droplets from bone marrow, or the release of catecholamine after trauma, which mobilizes fatty acids. Fat embolism can lodge in the lungs or even the brain and often occurs within 24 hours after the fracture, although it may be delayed up to 72 hours. Its typical symptoms include apprehension, sweating, fever, tachycardia, pallor, dyspnea, pulmonary effusion, tissue hypoxia, cyanosis, convulsions, and coma. The most distinctive sign, however, is a petechial rash on the chest and shoulders.

In fat embolism, arterial blood gas measurements show low PO_2, and chest X-ray may disclose a typical "snowstorm" pattern of infiltrates scattered over the lungs. Treatment consists of oxygen delivery by nasal catheter or mask, immobilization (if the fracture isn't already immobilized), and administration of heparin, corticosteroids, and a diuretic, such as furosemide, to reduce interstitial or pulmonary edema. Extensive pulmonary damage may require insertion of chest tubes, a tracheotomy, or use of a ventilator. Throughout treatment, monitor arterial blood gases and vital signs often.

Performing Pin Care

Once your patient has a pin in place—for skeletal traction or an external fixation device—the doctor will order pin care. Here are some general guidelines to follow:
• Examine the patient's skin around the pin for tautness, pain, tenderness, and redness from inflammation and infection.
• Note any crusted, serous drainage around the pin site. *Gently* remove the crust to prevent it from obstructing wound drainage.
• Give skin care every 4 hours.
• Note any signs and symptoms of pin looseness—such as increased or purulent drainage.
• Don't prod the patient's skin around the pin—you may cause additional pain or skin abrasions that can lead to infection.
• Clean the pins once or twice a day, using povidone-iodine or hydrogen peroxide, as ordered. For an external fixation device, work proximally to distally on one side, then on the other. Afterwards, wipe the device's frame with a sterile cloth moistened with sterile water and cover the pin ends.

Emergency Care of a Severed Body Part

Through microsurgery, reimplantation of a severed body part (such as a hand, foot, digit, or ear) may restore function as well as provide cosmetic repair. Crucial to the success of reimplantation is emergency care of the patient and the injured body part. The part must be wrapped and cooled quickly and properly, but need not be cleaned, to avoid further trauma. Irreversible tissue damage occurs after only 6 hours at ambient temperature. However, hypothermic management seldom preserves tissue for more than 24 hours.

To care for the patient with a severed body part:

• Make sure the hemorrhage at the amputation site is controlled.

• Place several sterile gauze sponges and an appropriate amount of sterile roller gauze in a sterile basin, and pour sterile normal saline solution or sterile lactated Ringer's solution over them. Put on sterile gloves.

• Place the moist gauze sponges over the stump; then wrap it with moist roller gauze. Put a watertight covering over the stump and place it in an ice-packed plastic bag. Avoid using dry ice *to prevent irreversible tissue damage.*

• Holding the body part in one hand, carefully cover it with the moist gauze sponges. Then wrap it with the moist roller gauze.

• Place the wrapped body part in a watertight plastic bag *to avoid contact between body tissue and ice, which can cause freezing and prevent reimplantation.* Tape the bag closed and put it in the ice-filled container. Label the container with the patient's name and identification number, as well as the date and time.

• Prepare the patient and the body part for transfer to a reimplantation center.

TRAUMATIC
EMERGENCIES

Initial Environmental Emergency Assessment Checklist

Assess the ABCs first and intervene appropriately.

CHECK FOR:

• wheezing or stridor, indicating laryngeal edema from anaphylaxis (due to bites or stings) or aspiration from near-drowning
• hypotension, indicating shock from hypothermia, hyperthermia, or a bite or sting
• increasing dyspnea, cough, stertorous respirations, and hemoptysis, indicating high-altitude pulmonary edema
• increasing headache, weakness, and altered level of consciousness, indicating high-altitude cerebral edema
• cyanosis, indicating hypoxemia in altitude-related illness, hypothermia, or near-drowning
• altered behavior and consciousness, indicating altitude-related illness, hypothermia, or hyperthermia
• dysrhythmias, indicating hyperkalemia, hypokalemia, or acidosis.

INTERVENE BY:

• administering 100% oxygen by face mask (warmed, if the patient's hypothermic)
• inserting a nasogastric or endotracheal tube (*except* in a patient with hypothermia, because vagal stimulation could cause ventricular fibrillation)
• starting an I.V. and administering fluids
• applying warm blankets or ice packs, as indicated.

PREPARE FOR:

• applying hypothermia or hyperthermia blankets
• beginning internal rewarming procedures, such as heated peritoneal, bladder, or gastric lavage
• administering antivenin, sodium bicarbonate, antiarrhythmics, or diuretics, as ordered
• taking a chest X-ray.

TRAUMATIC EMERGENCIES

Detecting Hypothermia

As you know, a patient's hypothermia may be very subtle; you may detect it only after taking his temperature. But if you always use a standard clinical thermometer, you still run the risk of overlooking hypothermia and of underestimating its severity. Why? Because most standard thermometers only register low temperatures to 94° F. (34.4° C.).

So, if you suspect that your patient has hypothermia (based on his history of exposure or immersion), be sure to take his temperature with a low-reading thermometer. Use a continuous-monitoring rectal probe, if possible. It has two important advantages: Rectal temperature most closely reflects core temperature, and you won't have to move your patient every 10 to 15 minutes to take manual rectal temperature readings.

Danger: Cold Blood

Strange as it may seem, your hypothermic patient's own blood can kill him if you don't take precautions while treating him. Why? Because the body responds to hypothermia by vasoconstriction, which shunts most of the blood to the core—the heart, lungs, and brain. The blood remaining in the extremities becomes very cold, acidotic, and hyperkalemic. If a sudden rush of this blood to the core occurs, it can cause ventricular fibrillation and death.

To avoid this, always take these precautions with a hypothermic patient:
• Handle him carefully at all times during treatment; keep him as still as possible, and don't allow him to exert himself in any way.
• Rewarm him both internally (with heated humidified oxygen or heated peritoneal dialysis) and externally (with hot packs or hot baths), as ordered.
• Question a doctor's order for any medication that will stimulate the patient's heart (such as atropine or epinephrine), unless you're *sure* he's in cardiac arrest.

Special Consideration

What happens in frostbite: The body's response to extremely cold temperatures is vasoconstriction. This decreases blood flow and oxygen supply to peripheral tissues as blood is shunted to the core. Thus deprived of oxygen, the peripheral tissues are especially susceptible to damage from cold.

Dealing with Frostbite

In most cases, you can recognize frostbite on a patient's arms, legs, or face by checking for the following: white or mottled blue-white skin that's hard to the touch, blisters, and complaints of numbness in the affected area.

Move the patient to a warm environment and cover him with blankets or additional clothing. Do not use electric blankets, hot water bottles, or heaters.

Handle the affected part gently, and protect it from friction and pressure. *Don't massage it*—this can cause tissue damage. If clothes are frozen to the area, don't try to remove them until after the area's thawed.

To thaw the frostbitten arm or leg, first immerse it in warm water (99° to 103° F. [37.2° to 39.4° C.]). If the affected area is on his face, apply moist, warm towels. Wait several minutes for the frozen area to thaw. As it does, the patient will regain sensation in that area and probably complain of severe pain. In addition, the affected area will look flushed and feel warm.

Discontinue the warm water immersion or towel applications. Administer tetanus toxoid and whatever sedatives or analgesics the doctor's ordered, checking first to make sure the patient's not allergic to them.

Look for other injuries, and find out if your patient has any chronic illnesses that may affect subsequent treatment.

Document the size and color of the affected area in your nurses' notes, as well as your care, information about his medical history, and the circumstances surrounding the injury.

Warn your patient and his family that he must be especially careful not to let the affected area get too cold in the future. Permanent tissue damage can result if previously frostbitten areas become frozen again.

Understanding Minor Heat-Related Illnesses

Except for heatstroke and heat exhaustion, heat-related illnesses generally aren't life-threatening. This chart will help you recognize and treat patients with these less serious disorders.

HEAT EDEMA

Signs and symptoms include mild swelling and a feeling of tightness in the hands and feet. Heat edema occurs in unacclimated persons—especially those who are elderly—during the first few days of heat exposure.

Treatment:
- Elevate the patient's extremities.
- Apply support hose, if necessary.
- No additional treatment's necessary; the edema is self-limiting and should resolve with acclimation.

HEAT TETANY

Carpopedal spasms (due to rapid changes in pH from hyperventilation) occur during overexposure to heat (heat tetany often accompanies heat exhaustion or heatstroke). Although a positive Chvostek's sign may be present, the patient's serum calcium level is normal.

Treatment:
- Move the patient to a cool environment.

- Heat tetany is self-limiting—it should resolve without treatment.

HEAT SYNCOPE

Signs and symptoms include brief lapses of consciousness from postural hypotension due to shunting of blood to dilated peripheral vessels. Water and salt depletion occur rarely.

Treatment:
- Place the patient in a supine position and elevate his legs.
- Hydrate him with oral fluids, if necessary.
- To prevent a recurrence, tell the patient to avoid sudden or prolonged standing in a hot environment.

HEAT CRAMPS

Painful cramps occur in the most strenuously used muscles (such as the thighs and shoulders) due to a decrease in extracellular sodium through sweating, dilution with free water, or both. Besides cramping, the patient may have nausea, cool and pallid skin, or diaphoresis.

Continued

Understanding Minor Heat-Related Illnesses
Continued

Treatment:
• To replace fluid and electrolytes, give the patient a balanced electrolyte drink, such as Gatorade.
• Loosen the patient's clothing, and have him lie down in a cool place.
• Massage his muscles. If his muscle cramps are severe, start an I.V. infusion with normal saline solution.

ANHIDROTIC HEAT EXHAUSTION

A poorly understood syndrome of weakness, polyuria, and failure of normal sweating, this syndrome often occurs after several months of heat acclimation and is usually preceded by prickly heat. Other signs and symptoms include tachycardia, tachypnea, and fever. Anhidrotic heat exhaustion predisposes the patient to heat stroke.

Treatment:
• Move the patient to a cool environment.
• Place him in a supine position and let him rest.
• Give him potassium supplements to replace the potassium lost through polyuria.
• Tell him to avoid strenuous physical activity until his condition improves.

How to Prevent Heat-Related Illnesses

Heat-related illnesses are easily preventable. As a nurse, you should educate the public to know how to prevent these illnesses. This information is especially vital for athletes involved in rigorous sports or for soldiers on maneuvers.
• Advise your patients to avoid heat by taking the following precautions in hot weather: wear loose-fitting, lightweight clothing; rest frequently; avoid hot places; and take in adequate fluids and electrolytes.
• Advise patients who are obese, elderly, or taking drugs that impair heat regulation to avoid overheating. Heat-related illness is often related to phenothiazines.
• Warn patients who have been treated for heat-related illnesses against going out in the sun again for awhile.

Guidelines for Tetanus Prophylaxis

Proper wound care *always* includes appropriate tetanus prophylaxis. To determine the correct immunization for your patient, you must know:
- his wound classification (tetanus-prone or non-tetanus-prone)
- his history of tetanus immunization.

First, use the chart below to classify your patient's wound. Then, after determining his history of tetanus immunization, use the immunization schedule on the right to identify the prophylaxis he'll need now.

WOUND CLASSIFICATION

CLINICAL FEATURES OF WOUND	TETANUS-PRONE WOUNDS	NON-TETANUS-PRONE WOUNDS
Age	Greater than 6 hours	Less than 6 hours
Configuration	Stellate wound, avulsion, abrasion	Linear wound
Depth	Greater than 1 cm (⅜")	Less than 1 cm (⅜")
Mechanism of injury	Missile, crush, burn, frostbite	Sharp surface (for example, a knife or a piece of glass)
Signs of infection	Present	Absent
Devitalized tissue	Present	Absent
Contaminants (for example, dirt, feces, soil, saliva)	Present	Absent
Denervated and/or ischemic tissue	Present	Absent

TRAUMATIC EMERGENCIES

Continued

Guidelines for Tetanus Prophylaxis
Continued

TETANUS PROPHYLAXIS

HISTORY OF TETANUS IMMUNIZATION (number of doses)	TETANUS-PRONE WOUNDS		NON-TETANUS-PRONE WOUNDS	
	Td*	TIG*	Td	TIG
Uncertain	Yes	Yes	Yes	No
0 to 1	Yes	Yes	Yes	No
2	Yes	No (*yes* if 24 hours since wound was inflicted)	Yes	No
3 or more	No (*yes* if more than 5 years since last dose)	No	No (*yes* if more than 10 years since last dose)	No

*Td = Tetanus and diphtheria toxoids absorbed (for adult use), 0.5 ml
**TIG = Tetanus immune globulin (human), 250 units
  When Td and TIG are given concurrently, separate syringes and separate sites should be used.
  Note: For children under age 7, diphtheria and tetanus toxoids and pertussis vaccine absorbed (D.P.T.) are preferred to tetanus toxoid alone. If pertussis vaccine is contraindicated, administer tetanus and diphtheria toxoids absorbed (D.T.).

Adapted from American College of Surgeons, Committee on Trauma, *Prophylaxis against Tetanus in Wound Management*, April 1984

TRAUMATIC EMERGENCIES

Initial Eye, Ear, Nose & Throat Assessment Checklist

Assess the ABCs first and intervene appropriately.

CHECK FOR:

• decreased sensation, facial asymmetry, limited extraocular movements, and hearing or vision loss, indicating possible neuromuscular damage
• local swelling, redness, drainage, fever, tenderness, and lesions, indicating possible infection
• nasal or neck swelling and stridor, dyspnea, or tachypnea, indicating respiratory compromise.

INTERVENE BY:

• administering supplemental oxygen by nasal cannula or mask
• applying ice packs
• irrigating your patient's eyes
• administering eye medication.

PREPARE FOR:

• eye protection
• intraocular pressure testing
• visual acuity and hearing testing
• fluorescein staining
• nasal packing
• carbogen therapy
• ear irrigation.

Understanding Fluorescein Staining

Fluorescein staining of a patient's eye helps the doctor detect foreign bodies, corneal abrasions, or other corneal injuries.

Fluorescein dye applied to the patient's palpebral conjunctiva temporarily turns the sclera orange. Then, when the doctor shines a cobalt blue light on the eye, damaged epithelium shows up as bright green, indicating a corneal injury.

Use fluorescein strips instead of drops, which can easily become contaminated with *Pseudomonas*. After staining your patient's eye, have him gently roll his eyes with his lids closed so the dye spreads over his cornea. After the examination, irrigate his eye with normal saline solution to remove the excess dye.

Pediatric EENT Emergencies

FOREIGN BODY IN THE NOSE

When a child inserts an object into his nose, the foul-smelling discharge that results alarms the parents, who bring the child to the doctor.

Ask the child if he's put something up his nose. Then explain that you're going to help him. Tell the parent that an otolaryngologist will remove the object easily, if it's visible, with a nasal speculum and bayonet forceps, Fogarty catheter, or suction forceps.

Depending on the child's age, he may have to be restrained with an Olympic papoose or a blanket wrapped around him. Let the parents help you, unless they're apt to become frightened or anxious.

If the doctor can't see the foreign body in the nose, he may insert cocaine packs to anesthetize the area, shrink mucous membranes, and facilitate examination. After removal, the doctor may prescribe antibiotics.

FOREIGN BODY IN THE EAR

If a child is brought to the ED with an object in his ear, you'll probably have to restrain him before you can remove it. Tell the child how you're going to help him. Then use a Pedi-wrap, an Olympic papoose, or a blanket wrapped around the child to keep him still. Position his head and hold it firmly in place.

The doctor will use angled forceps or "alligator" forceps to remove the object. Or he may use a suction tip or a suction cup.

If the object is difficult to remove, the doctor will anesthetize the child first to alleviate his pain and anxiety. Antibiotic ear drops may be ordered to prevent infection.

TRAUMATIC EMERGENCIES

Guide to Common EENT Emergencies

CORNEAL ABRASION, CORNEAL ULCER

Signs and symptoms:
- Severe eye pain
- Excessive tearing
- Reddened conjunctiva
- Squinting
- Photophobia
- History of eye trauma or eye infection

Nursing considerations:
- Administer topical anesthetic, if ordered. Make sure your patient's not allergic to it.
- Examine the affected eye with a flashlight. If no lesion's visible but you strongly suspect one, call the doctor. He may instill fluorescein sodium (Flu-Glo Strips*) and examine the eye under a slit lamp or ultraviolet light. Irrigate your patient's eye with artificial tears after the exam.
- If examination reveals a corneal abrasion or ulcer, the doctor may ask you to instill antibiotic ointment and apply an eye patch.
- Apply warm compresses to the affected eye, if ordered, to help relieve discomfort. Be sure your patient's eye is closed *before* you apply a compress to it.
- Give oral medication for pain, if ordered.
- To help relieve photophobia, instruct your patient to wear dark glasses.

ACTINIC TRAUMA (WELDER'S FLASH)

Signs and symptoms:
- History of overexposure to sunlight, ultraviolet light source (sunlamp), welding arc, or germicidal lamp
- Severe eye pain that may begin several hours after exposure

Nursing considerations:
- Instill anesthetic eye drops, antibiotic ointment, or antibiotic eye drops in affected eye, as ordered. Apply patches to both eyes. *Note:* The doctor may order eye patches to remain in place for 24 hours. Make sure your patient can get home safely and won't be left alone during the 24-hour period.
- Give analgesic, as ordered. Reassure your patient that his eye pain probably won't last longer than 24 hours.
- Instruct your patient to see an ophthalmologist for a follow-up examination, if pain persists. Otherwise, your patient can remove the eye patches and resume normal activities.

Continued

Guide to Common EENT Emergencies
Continued

LACERATION OF THE EYEBALL

Signs and symptoms:
- Severe eye pain; poor vision
- External leakage of ocular fluid
- Embedded foreign body
- Blood in anterior chamber of eye
- History of recent blow to the eye or an injury to surrounding tissue

Nursing considerations:
- Call the doctor immediately.
- Reassure your patient, and instruct him to lie flat until the doctor arrives. Meanwhile, apply an eye shield to help protect the affected eye. Don't permit the shield to press on the eyeball.
- Get a detailed history of the injury. Include the time of the accident, as well as how it occurred.
- Avoid touching the patient's eye during the examination. Use very *light pressure,* or you'll cause further injury.
- Administer a sedative, as ordered, and prepare your patient for surgery, if his condition requires it.

PERFORATED EARDRUM

Signs and symptoms:
- Severe ear pain, possibly followed by a sudden decrease in pain as the eardrum ruptures

- Ear drainage
- Fever
- Possible bleeding
- Burns in or surrounding ear

Nursing considerations:
- Reassure your patient. Have an otoscope ready, and assist the doctor with ear exam.
- Get patient's complete medical history.
- If perforation is caused by penetrating object, have tweezers available to remove any imbedded particles. Never irrigate the ear.
- If burns are present, give burn care as needed.
- Give antibiotic ear drops, as ordered.
- Instruct your patient to keep his ear clean and dry. Tell him to place a cotton ball or ear mold inside his outer ear when showering or shampooing.

EPISTAXIS

Signs and symptoms:
- Frank bleeding from nose
- Restlessness; anxiety, apprehension; cool, clammy skin; rapid, thready pulse; low blood pressure
- Pale mucous membranes in nasal passage
- History of nasal injury, recent upper respiratory infection, hypertension, blood dyscrasia, coronary artery disease, or alcoholism

Continued

Guide to Common EENT Emergencies
Continued

EPISTAXIS
Continued

Nursing considerations:
● Take the patient's history. Find out if he's taking any medications. Look for Medic Alert bracelet to see if he has blood dyscrasia.
● With blood dyscrasia, the doctor may order vitamin K,* and plasma.
● Place patient in seated position. Instruct him to pinch his nose shut with 4" x 4" sterile gauze pads. Bend his head forward slightly so he won't swallow any blood. If that's unsuccessful, apply ice to back of his neck.
● Gather: a nasal speculum; a suction device, with angulated nasal tip; cocaine strips; electrocautery apparatus; silver nitrate sticks; and leads from chromic acid beads.
● If the doctor can't stop the bleeding, he may want you to help insert a nasal pack.

FRACTURED TOOTH

Signs and symptoms:
● If tooth enamel is involved, the fracture site will be rough but not sensitive to touch.
● If the dentin is exposed, the tooth may be sensitive to touch or air. The color of the fracture surface will be yellowish-brown.

● If the fracture has exposed the pulp, the tooth will appear pink. It will be painful when touched.
● If the root is involved, the tooth will be loose. It will be painful when tooth is touched.
Nursing considerations:
● Gather the following equipment: dental burs, stone or sandpaper disks.
● If dentin is involved, cover the fractured area with a clean 2" x 2" sterile gauze pad. Administer pain medication, as ordered.
● If pulp is exposed, place a sedative dressing on the exposed area, per doctor's order. Prepare for dentist to perform partial pulpotomy or pulpectomy, if necessary.

FRACTURED LARYNX

Signs and symptoms:
● Severe face and neck pain
● Anterior cervical neck area appears flat
● Subcutaneous emphysema over larynx
● Nonpalpable thyroid cartilage
● Dysphagia and hoarseness
Nursing considerations:
● Don't leave patient. Reassure him.
● Be alert for possible airway obstruction. Have trach set and suction equipment ready. Doctor may perform bedside tracheotomy.

TRAUMATIC EMERGENCIES

*Available in the United States and Canada.

Continued

Guide to Common EENT Emergencies
Continued

FRACTURED LARYNX
Continued

• Always look for laryngeal trauma or fracture in a patient with multiple injuries. Remember, a halter seat belt can cause fractured larynx in a car accident victim.

ACUTE EPIGLOTTITIS

Signs and symptoms:
• Dyspnea or apnea in severe cases

• High fever
• Inspiratory stridor in children (rarely heard in adults)
• Severe sore throat, with cherry-red, enlarged epiglottis
• Possible substernal retraction on inspiration
• Coughing and hoarseness
Nursing considerations:
• Make sure patient has an open airway. If he's in a seated position, thrust his chest forward and hyperextend his neck.
• Be prepared to assist doctor if he wants to intubate patient or do an emergency tracheotomy.
• Be prepared to start appropriate I.V. therapy with antibiotics and steroids, per doctor's orders.

How to Apply an Eye Patch

Your patient may need an eye patch to prevent contamination, to discourage eye movement, and to promote healing. The next time you're asked to apply an eye patch, keep the following pointers in mind:
• Use as many gauze pads as you need to fill the orbital depth so the patch is level with the patient's frontal edge.

• Tape the patch diagonally from the medial orbital rim to the lateral cheekbone. (Remember to use paper tape so you won't irritate your patient's skin when you remove the patch later.)
• After you've applied the patch, ask your patient to try to open his eye. He shouldn't be able to do this if the patch is of the right depth and correctly placed.

TRAUMATIC
EMERGENCIES

Classification of Penicillin Reactions

STAGE	REACTION TIME	SIGNS AND SYMPTOMS
I. Immediate (most dangerous)	Within 30 minutes	Urticaria, systemic anaphylaxis
II. Accelerated	Within 2 to 72 hours	Pruritus, urticaria, wheezing, laryngeal edema, local inflammatory reactions
III. Late (most common: 80% to 90%)	After 72 hours (sometimes weeks later)	Morbilliform, urticarial, and erythematous eruptions; serum sickness; local inflammatory reactions

Highlighting Epinephrine in Anaphylactic Shock

Although epinephrine is the drug of choice in treating anaphylactic shock, if you give your patient even a slight overdose or infuse the drug too rapidly, he may develop cardiac dysrhythmias and a sudden rise in blood pressure. So observe the following guidelines when administering epinephrine to your patient:
• Use epinephrine cautiously in patients with angina, dysrhythmias, or hyperthyroid conditions.
• Administer epinephrine by subcutaneous (S.C.) injection unless your patient's in profound shock or refractory to S.C. injection. I.V. epinephrine can be given by slow bolus or infusion. I.M. injection is also possible; however, impaired absorption may occur. Endotracheal tube administration is a last resort for a patient in severe shock who doesn't have an accessible I.V. line.
• Start with a small dose, and repeat it every 10 minutes until your patient stabilizes.
• Check your patient's vital signs frequently and, if possible, continuously monitor his cardiac rhythm.

Guide to Commonly Abused Substances

AMPHETAMINES

• amphetamine sulfate (Benzedrine)—bennies, greenies, cartwheels
• methamphetamine (Methadrin)—speed, meth, crystal
• dextroamphetamine sulfate (Dexedrine)—dexies, hearts, oranges

Signs and symptoms:
• Dilated reactive pupils
• Altered mental status (from confusion to paranoia)
• Hallucinations
• Tremors and seizure activity
• Hyperactive tendon reflexes
• Exhaustion
• Coma
• Dry mouth
• Shallow respirations
• Tachycardia
• Hypertension
• Hyperthermia
• Diaphoresis

Assessment and intervention:
• If the drug was taken orally, induce vomiting or perform gastric lavage; give activated charcoal and a sodium or magnesium sulfate cathartic, as ordered.
• Acidify the patient's urine by adding ammonium chloride or ascorbic acid to his I.V. solution, as ordered, to lower his urine pH to 5.
• Force diuresis by giving the patient mannitol, as ordered.

• Expect to give a short-acting barbiturate, such as pentobarbital, to control stimulant-induced seizure activity.
• Restrain the patient to keep him from injuring himself and others—especially if he's paranoid or hallucinating.
• Give *haloperidol (Haldol)* I.M., as ordered, to treat agitation or assaultive behavior.
• Give an alpha-adrenergic blocking agent, such as *phentolamine (Regitine),* for hypertension, as ordered.
• Watch for cardiac dysrhythmias. Notify the doctor if these develop, and expect to give *propanolol* or *lidocaine* to treat tachydysrhythmias or ventricular dysrhythmias, respectively.
• Treat hyperthermia with tepid sponge baths or a hypothermia blanket, as ordered.
• Provide a quiet environment to avoid overstimulation.
• Be alert for signs and symptoms of withdrawal, such as abdominal tenderness, muscle aches, and long periods of sleep.
• Observe suicide precautions, especially if the patient shows signs of withdrawal.

Continued

Guide to Commonly Abused Substances
Continued

COCAINE

- "free-base"
- cocaine hydrochloride

Signs and symptoms:
- Dilated pupils
- Confusion
- Alternating euphoria/apprehension
- Hyperexcitability
- Visual, auditory, and olfactory hallucinations
- Spasms and seizure activity
- Coma
- Tachypnea
- Hyperpnea
- Pallor or cyanosis
- Respiratory arrest
- Tachycardia
- Hypertension/hypotension
- Fever
- Nausea and vomiting
- Abdominal pain
- Perforated nasal septum or oral sores

Assessment and intervention:
- Calm the patient down by talking to him in a quiet room.
- If cocaine was ingested, induce vomiting or perform gastric lavage; give activated charcoal followed by a saline cathartic, as ordered.
- Give the patient a tepid sponge bath and administer an antipyretic, as ordered, to reduce fever.
- Monitor his blood pressure and heart rate. Expect to give *propranolol* for symptomatic tachycardia.
- Administer an anticonvulsant, such as *diazepam (Valium)*, as ordered, to control seizure activity.
- Scrape the inside of his nose to remove residual amounts of the drug.
- Monitor his cardiac rate and rhythm—ventricular fibrillation and cardiac standstill can occur as a direct cardiotoxic result of cocaine. Defibrillate and initiate CPR, if indicated.

HALLUCINOGENS

- lysergic acid diethylamide (LSD)—hawk, acid, sunshine
- mescaline (peyote)— mese, cactus, big chief

Signs and symptoms:
- Dilated pupils
- Intensified perceptions
- Agitation and anxiety
- Synesthesia
- Impaired judgment
- Hyperactive movement
- Flashback experiences
- Hallucinations
- Depersonalization
- Moderately increased blood pressure

Continued

TRAUMATIC EMERGENCIES

Guide to Commonly Abused Substances
Continued

HALLUCINOGENS *Continued*

- Increased heart rate
- Fever
- Blank staring
- Nystagmus
- Amnesia
- Decreased awareness of surroundings
- Recurrent coma
- Violent behavior
- Hyperactivity
- Seizure activity
- Gait ataxia
- Muscle rigidity
- Drooling
- Hyperthermia
- Hypertensive crisis
- Cardiac arrest

Assessment and intervention:
- Reorient the patient repeatedly to time, place, and person.
- Restrain the patient to protect him from injuring himself and others.
- Calm the patient down by talking to him in a quiet room.
- If the drug was taken orally, induce vomiting or perform gastric lavage; give charcoal and a cathartic, as ordered.
- Give *Valium* I.V., as ordered, to control seizure activity.

HALLUCINOGENS

- phencyclidine (PCP)—angel dust, peace pill, hog

Signs and symptoms:
- *See signs and symptoms listed under lysergic acid diethylamide and mescaline, beginning on p. 162.*

Assessment and intervention:
- If the drug was taken orally, induce vomiting or perform gastric lavage; instill and remove activated charcoal repeatedly, as ordered.
- Force acidic diuresis by acidifying the patient's urine with ascorbic acid, as ordered, to increase excretion of the drug.
- Expect to continue to acidify his urine for 2 weeks.
- Give *Valium* and *Haldol,* as ordered, to control agitation or psychotic behavior.
- Administer diazepam, as ordered, to control seizure activity.
- Provide a quiet environment and dimmed light.
- Give *propranolol (Inderal),* as ordered, to treat hypertension and tachycardia. If the patient's hypertension is severe, give nitroprusside, as ordered.
- Closely monitor his urine output and serial renal function tests—rhabdomyolysis, myoglobinuria, and renal failure may occur in severe intoxication.
- If the patient develops renal failure, prepare him for hemodialysis.

Continued

TRAUMATIC
EMERGENCIES

Guide to Commonly Abused Substances
Continued

ALCOHOL (ETHANOL)

- beer and wine
- distilled spirits
- other preparations, such as cough syrup, after-shave, or mouthwash
Signs and symptoms:
- Ataxia
- Seizure activity
- Coma
- Hypothermia
- Alcohol breath odor
- Respiratory depression
- Bradycardia
- Hypotension
- Nausea and vomiting
Assessment and intervention:
- Expect to induce vomiting or perform gastric lavage if ingestion occurred in the previous 4 hours. Give activated charcoal and a saline cathartic, as ordered.
- Start I.V. fluid replacement and administer dextrose, thiamine, B-complex vitamins, and Vitamin C, as ordered, to prevent dehydration and hypoglycemia and to correct nutritional deficiencies.
- Pad bed rails and apply cloth restraints to protect the patient from injury.
- Give an anticonvulsant such as diazepam, as ordered, to control seizure activity.

TRAUMATIC EMERGENCIES

- Watch the patient for signs and symptoms of withdrawal, such as hallucinations and delirium tremens. If these occur, give *chlordiazepoxide (Librium), chloral hydrate,* or *paraldehyde,* as ordered. (Be sure to administer paraldehyde with a glass syringe or glass cup to avoid a chemical reaction with plastic.)
- Auscultate the patient's lungs frequently to detect rales or rhonchi, possibly indicating aspiration pneumonia. If you note these breath sounds, expect to give antibiotics.
- Perform neurologic assessments, and monitor the patient's vital signs every 15 minutes until he's stable.
- Assist with dialysis if the patient's vital functions are severely depressed.

BARBITURATE SEDATIVES/ HYPNOTICS

- barbiturates—downers, sleepers, barbs
- amobarbital sodium (Amytal sodium)—blue angels, blue devils, bluebirds
- phenobarbital (Luminal)—phennies, purple hearts, goofballs
- secobarbital sodium (Seconal)—reds, red devils, seccy

Continued

Guide to Commonly Abused Substances
Continued

BARBITURATE SEDATIVES/
HYPNOTICS
Continued

Signs and symptoms:
• Poor pupil reaction to light
• Nystagmus
• Depressed level of consciousness (from confusion to coma)
• Flaccid muscles and absent reflexes
• Hyperthermia or hypothermia
• Cyanosis
• Respiratory depression
• Hypotension
• Blisters or bullous lesions
Assessment and intervention:
• Induce vomiting or perform gastric lavage if the patient ingested the drug within last 4 hours; give activated charcoal and a saline cathartic, as ordered.
• Maintain his blood pressure with I.V. fluid challenges and vasopressors, as ordered.
• If the patient's taken a phenobarbital overdose, give *sodium bicarbonate* I.V., as ordered.
• Use a hyper- or hypothermia blanket, as ordered, to help normalize the patient's temperature.
• Prepare your patient for hemodialysis or hemoperfusion if toxicity is severe.
• Perform frequent neurologic assessments and check your patient's pulse rate, temperature, skin color, and reflexes often.

• Notify the doctor if you see signs of respiratory distress or pulmonary edema.
• Watch for signs of withdrawal, such as hyperreflexia, grand mal seizures, and hallucinations.
• Protect the patient from injuring himself and provide symptomatic relief of withdrawal symptoms, as ordered.

NARCOTICS

• heroin—smack, H, junk, snow
• morphine—mort, monkey, M, Miss Emma
• hydromorphone hydrochloride (Dilaudid)— D, lords
Signs and symptoms:
• Constricted pupils
• Depressed level of consciousness (but the patient's usually responsive to persistent verbal or tactile stimuli)
• Seizure activity
• Hypothermia
• Slow, deep respirations
• Hypotension
• Bradycardia
• Skin changes (pruritus, urticaria, and flushed skin)
Assessment and intervention:
• Repeat *naloxone (Narcan)* administration, as ordered, until the drug's CNS depressant effects are reversed.
• Replace fluids I.V., as ordered, to increase circulatory volume.

TRAUMATIC
EMERGENCIES

Continued

Guide to Commonly Abused Substances
Continued

NARCOTICS
Continued

• Correct hypothermia by applying extra blankets; if the patient's body temperature doesn't increase, use a hyperthermia blanket, as ordered.
• Reorient the patient frequently.
• Auscultate his lungs frequently for rales, possibly indicating pulmonary edema. (Onset may be delayed.)

• Administer oxygen via nasal cannula, mask, or mechanical ventilation to correct hypoxemia from hypoventilation.
• Monitor cardiac rate and rhythm, being alert for atrial fibrillation. (This should resolve spontaneously when the hypoxemia's corrected.)
• Be alert for signs of withdrawal, such as piloerection (goose flesh), diaphoresis, and hyperactive bowel sounds.

Assessing Drug Use

With *all* types of drug abuse, your assessment of the patient's drug use pattern is critical. Find out:
• what drugs the patient is using.
• how much he uses and how often.
• how long he has been using them.
  Remember, such a patient may be unwilling or unable to give you a history of his drug use. So collect further information by talking with his family or friends, by physical examination, and by blood and urine tests. Be alert for accompanying disorders since these also require treatment.

TRAUMATIC
EMERGENCIES

First Aid for Bite Victims

Animal bites:
Immediately wash the bite vigorously with soap and water for at least 10 minutes to remove the animal's saliva. As soon as possible, flush the wound with a viricidal agent, followed by a clear-water rinse. After cleansing the wound, apply a sterile dressing. If possible, don't suture the wound, and don't immediately stop the bleeding (unless it's massive), since blood flow helps to cleanse the wound.

Question the patient about the animal bite. Ask if he provoked the animal (if so, chances are it's not rabid) and if he can identify it or its owner (since the animal may need to be confined for observation).

Black widow spider bites:
Black widow spider bites may go unnoticed until severe pain at the puncture site and intense, cramping abdominal pain strike the victim 10 to 40 minutes later. Since no lab test can detect the cause, a diagnosis must be made clinically. When taking a history, ask the patient if he's recently been in a lumber or junk pile, an outdoor privy, or an old barn, garage, or basement. Black widow spiders may inhabit any of these places.

Spider bite victims may suffer spasmodic muscle pain in the legs, chest, and back. At the puncture site you'll see two tiny red spots and slight swelling or urticaria. The patient will experience weakness, nausea, fever, chills, and a rigid abdomen with diminished bowel sounds. He'll have elevated blood pressure, labored breathing, profuse sweating, and numb or tingling feet. Small children may suffer delirium and convulsions.

Keep the patient quiet and the affected part immobile. If a tourniquet is in place, check his pulse regularly. Don't release the tourniquet as this would also release toxins into the circulatory system. Apply cold packs to relieve pain and swelling and to slow circulation.

Snake bites
Poisonous snakes inhabit every state in the United States except Hawaii, Alaska, and Maine. Even though snakebite victims represent a small percentage of ED cases, be prepared to act quickly in such an emergency.

Snakebite victims commonly arrive at the ED with a tourniquet tied tightly around the affected extremity. If so, don't remove the tourniquet as this would release the venom suddenly into the patient's system.

Call the doctor, maintain a patent airway, and begin I.V. fluids. The doctor will prescribe antivenin and oxygen. Keep the patient quiet and the affected part immobile.

TRAUMATIC EMERGENCIES

Guidelines for Rabies Prophylaxis

When caring for a victim of an animal bite, don't forget to assess his need for rabies prophylaxis. As you know, untreated rabies is invariably fatal—so take every precaution to protect your patient. This chart contains the information you'll need.

If rabies prophylaxis is indicated, give your patient both rabies immune globin (RIG) and human diploid cell rabies vaccine (HDCV) *immediately*, as ordered. If RIG isn't available, expect to administer antirabies serum, equine.

ANIMAL	CONDITION OF ANIMAL AT TIME OF ATTACK	RABIES PROPHYLAXIS
Domestic (dog, cat)	Healthy and available for 10 days of observation	None, unless animal develops rabies during observation*
	Rabid or suspected rabid	RIG and HDCV
	Unknown (escaped)	Consult public health officials; if treatment's indicated, give RIG and HDCV
Wild (raccoon, skunk, bat, fox, and other carnivores)	*Consider all rabid unless proven negative by laboratory tests on captured animals**	RIG and HDCV
Others (livestock, rodents, and rabbits)	Consider individually; consult public health officials. Rodent and rabbit bites rarely cause rabies in humans.	Consult public health officials

* During the 10-day holding period, begin treating your patient with RIG and HDCV at the first sign of rabies in the animal, when the animal should be killed and tested immediately.
** The animal should be killed and tested as soon as possible; holding it for observation delays your patient's treatment (if needed).

Adapted from "Rabies Prevention," *Morbidity, Mortality Weekly Report*, 29:279, 1980.

TRAUMATIC
EMERGENCIES

Initial Metabolic and Endocrine Emergency Assessment Checklist

Assess the ABCs first and intervene appropriately.

CHECK FOR:

- wheezing or stridor, indicating airway obstruction from laryngeal spasm related to hypocalcemia from hypoparathyroidism
- tachypnea, indicating hypermetabolism, such as in thyrotoxic crisis; bradypnea, indicating hypometabolism, such as in myxedema coma; or Kussmaul's respirations, indicating diabetic ketoacidosis (DKA)
- alterations in level of consciousness, indicating DKA, hyperglycemic hyperosmolar nonketotic coma (HHNC), or hypoglycemia
- dry mucous membranes, dry skin, and decreased skin turgor, indicating severe dehydration from DKA, HHNC, or adrenal crisis
- decreased blood pressure, increased pulse rate, and cool, clammy skin, indicating hypovolemia such as in DKA, HHNC, or adrenal crisis.

INTERVENE BY:

- inserting a large-bore I.V. line and administering fluids, as ordered.

PREPARE FOR:

- an EKG tracing to check for dysrhythmias and electrolyte imbalances
- administration of glucose, potassium, sodium bicarbonate, or other electrolytes, and hormones.

Nursing Tip

Special Note: Remember to *suspect* an endocrine emergency whenever you see an obviously sick, distressed patient with an altered level of consciousness and signs of increased or decreased metabolism.

NONTRAUMATIC EMERGENCIES

Dealing with Metabolic Acidosis

Metabolic acidosis is a state of *excess* acid accumulation and *deficient* bicarbonate (base) in the blood, resulting from conditions that cause:
- excessive fat metabolism in the absence of carbohydrates
- anaerobic metabolism
- underexcretion of metabolized acids or inability to conserve base
- loss of sodium bicarbonate from the intestines.

Arterial pH level is below 7.35; HCO_3 is below 22 mEq/liter.

PREDISPOSING FACTORS

- DKA
- Addison's disease
- Renal failure
- Starvation
- Ethanol intoxication
- Tissue hypoxia
- Diarrhea
- Intestinal malabsorption
- Salicylate poisoning
- Low-carbohydrate, high-fat diet

SIGNS AND SYMPTOMS

- Headache and lethargy
- Central nervous system depression that may progress to coma
- Cardiac dysrhythmias
- Nausea and vomiting
- Anorexia
- Dehydration
- Kussmaul's respirations (a sign that respiratory compensation's beginning)

COMPENSATION

In the presence of low HCO_3, the respiratory system compensates with *hyperventilation* to *decrease* H_2CO_3 (as reflected in PCO_2) and to bring pH to normal by adjusting the ratio of HCO_3 to H_2CO_3 to 20:1 (normal).

INTERVENTIONS

- Give the patient sodium bicarbonate I.V.
- Evaluate and correct his electrolyte imbalances.
- Observe precautions to prevent seizures.
- Monitor his vital signs and fluid balance.
- Treat the underlying cause, as ordered.

Dealing with Metabolic Alkalosis

In contrast to metabolic acidosis, metabolic alkalosis is a state of *decreased* acid and *increased* bicarbonate (base) in the blood, resulting from conditions that cause:
- severe acid loss
- decreased serum potassium and chloride
- excessive bicarbonate intake.

Arterial pH level is above 7.45; HCO_3 is above 29 mEq/liter.

PREDISPOSING FACTORS

- Vomiting
- GI suctioning
- Diuretic therapy
- Corticosteroid therapy
- Cushing's syndrome
- Excessive bicarbonate intake
- Hypokalemia
- Hypercalcemia

SIGNS AND SYMPTOMS

- Neuromuscular irritability
- Tetany
- Twitching
- Seizures
- Central nervous system depression that may progress to coma
- Cardiac dysrhythmias
- Nausea and vomiting
- Hypoventilation (a sign that respiratory compensation's beginning)

COMPENSATION

In the presence of high HCO_3, the respiratory system compensates with *hypoventilation* to *increase* H_2CO_3 (as reflected in PCO_2) and to bring pH to normal by adjusting the ratio of HCO_3 to H_2CO_3 to 20:1 (normal).

INTERVENTIONS

- Give the patient normal saline solution and potassium I.V.
- Evaluate and correct his electrolyte imbalances.
- If his alkalosis is severe, give ammonium chloride I.V.
- Observe precautions to prevent seizures.
- Monitor his vital signs and fluid balance.
- Discontinue diuretics, if previously given.
- Treat the underlying cause, as ordered.

Guide to Life-Threatening Diabetic Complications

COMPLICATIONS	SYMPTOMS
Diabetic ketoacidosis (DKA)	Anorexia, nausea, vomiting, polyuria, weakness, malaise, dry skin, fruity-smelling (acetone) breath, Kussmaul's respirations, abdominal pain, hyperglycemia (blood glucose from 400 to 800 mg/100 ml); if untreated, may lead to drowsiness, stupor, coma
Hyperglycemic hyperosmolar nonketotic coma (HHNC)	Vomiting, diarrhea, tachycardia, hypotension, rapid breathing, flushed appearance, dry mucous membranes, volume depletion, alterations in levels of consciousness, focal motor seizures, transient hemiplegia, severe hyperglycemia (blood glucose about 1,000 mg/100 ml), possibly leading to stupor, coma
Insulin shock (hypoglycemia)	Sweating; tremors; increased blood pressure, pulse rate, respirations; headache; confusion; incoordination; blood glucose 50 mg/100 ml or less; may lead to convulsions, coma

NONTRAUMATIC EMERGENCIES

CAUSE	INSULIN LEVELS	MORTALITY
• Cessation of insulin, or physical or emotional stress • Occurs predominantly in Type I diabetes (insulin-dependent)	Zero	In known diabetics, approximately 5% (most commonly due to late treatment)
• Drugs (steroids, diuretics) • Infection • Major burns treated with high concentrations of sugar • Stress • Severe dehydration from sustained hyperglycemic diuresis, in which patient cannot sustain adequate fluid levels • Occurs predominantly in Type II diabetes (non-insulin-dependent)	Low (some residual ability to secrete insulin)	About 50%; treatment may be complicated by patient's age and debilitated state
• Too much insulin, too little food, excessive physical activity	High	Prognosis satisfactory when treated immediately; prolonged hypoglycemia can lead to permanent central nervous system damage

Initial Hematologic Emergency Assessment Checklist

Assess the ABCs first and intervene appropriately.

CHECK FOR:

- petechiae, ecchymoses, hematoma, or uncontrolled bleeding, indicating a coagulation disorder
- fever, chills, subnormal body temperature, or signs of dehydration, possibly indicating sepsis
- progressively deteriorating mental status, possibly indicating cerebral ischemia due to red blood cell sickling
- shortness of breath, tachypnea, or cyanosis, indicating hypoxemia from decreased red blood cells.

INTERVENE BY:

- inserting a large-gauge I.V. for fluid or blood component therapy
- applying thrombin-soaked gauze or Gelfoam to bleeding sites to promote coagulation and hemostasis.

PREPARE FOR:

- blood or component transfusion or factor replacement
- reverse isolation.

What Happens in Hemophilia

Hemophilia A and B are genetically transmitted clotting disorders caused by coagulation-factor deficiencies. Hemophilia A (classic hemophilia) is more common and results from a Factor VIII deficiency; hemophilia B results from Factor IX deficiency. Normal amounts of these factors circulate in both types of hemophilia, but they're functionally inadequate.

Once injury occurs, the clotting factor deficiency disrupts normal clotting by stopping Factor X activation, prothrombin-thrombin conversion, and fibrinogen-fibrin conversion. The end result:

impaired clot formation and continued bleeding at the injury site.

Hemophilia A and B are sex-linked (X chromosome), recessive traits. Males with the abnormal chromosome have the disorder and can transmit the gene. Females can be carriers but don't have the characteristic effects. Each daughter of a *carrier* has a 50% chance of being a carrier; each son of a carrier has a 50% chance of having the disorder. If a *hemophiliac* has children, all of his daughters will be carriers, but none of his sons will have the disorder.

Recognizing Transfusion Reactions

During a blood transfusion, your patient's at risk for developing any of five types of reactions. To learn to recognize them and to intervene appropriately, study this chart.

If your patient develops any sign or symptom of a reaction, immediately follow this procedure:
- Stop the transfusion
- Change the I.V. tubing to prevent infusing any more blood. Save the tubing and blood bag for analysis.
- Administer saline solution I.V. to keep the vein open.
- Take the patient's vital signs.
- Notify the doctor.
- Obtain urine and blood samples from the patient and send them to the laboratory.
- Prepare for further treatment.

REACTION	SIGNS AND SYMPTOMS	NURSING CONSIDERATIONS
Hemolytic	Include chills, fever, low back pain, headache, chest pain, tachycardia, dyspnea, hypotension, nausea and vomiting, restlessness, anxiety, shock	• Expect to place the patient in a supine position, with his legs elevated 20° to 30°, and to administer oxygen, fluids, and epinephrine to correct shock. • Expect to administer mannitol to maintain renal circulation. • Expect to insert an indwelling (Foley) catheter to monitor urinary output (should be about 100 ml/hr). • Expect to administer antipyretics to lower fever. If the fever persists, expect to apply a hypothermal blanket or to give tepid sponge or alcohol baths.

Continued

Recognizing Transfusion Reactions
Continued

REACTION	SIGNS AND SYMPTOMS	NURSING CONSIDERATIONS
Plasma protein incompatibility	Include chills, fever, flushing, abdominal pain, diarrhea, dyspnea, hypotension	• Expect to place the patient in a supine position, with his legs elevated 20° to 30°, and to administer oxygen, fluids, and epinephrine to correct shock. • Expect to administer corticosteroids.
Blood contamination	Include chills, fever, abdominal pain, nausea and vomiting, bloody diarrhea, hypotension	• Expect to administer fluids, antibiotics, corticosteroids, vasopressors, and a fresh transfusion.
Febrile	Range from mild chills, flushing, and fever to extreme signs and symptoms resembling a hemolytic reaction	• Expect to administer an antipyretic and an antihistamine for a *mild* reaction. • Expect to treat a *severe* reaction the same as a hemolytic reaction.
Allergic	Range from pruritus, urticaria, hives, facial swelling, chills, fever, nausea and vomiting, headache, and wheezing to laryngeal edema, respiratory distress, and shock	• Expect to administer parenteral antihistamines or, for a severe reaction, epinephrine or corticosteroids. • If the patient's only sign of reaction is hives, expect to restart the infusion, as ordered, at a slower rate.

Initial Poisoning Assessment Checklist

Assess the ABCs first and intervene appropriately.

CHECK PATIENT FOR:

• hypoactivity, decreased level of consciousness, bradycardia, or decreased respiratory rate, suggesting central nervous system (CNS) depression
• hyperactivity, tachycardia, tachypnea, or hyperventilation, suggesting CNS stimulation
• needle tracks, possibly indicating drug injection
• circumoral blisters or crystal residue, possibly indicating corrosive substance ingestion; blisters or erythema on the skin, possibly indicating barbiturate, carbon monoxide, or glutethimide poisoning; or powdered residue on the patient's skin or clothing, possibly from an insecticide.

INTERVENE BY:

• inducing vomiting with ipecac syrup or performing gastric lavage
• starting an I.V. and giving dextrose 50% in water, thiamine, and naloxone (Narcan), as ordered, if the patient's unresponsive
• administering activated charcoal and cathartics, as ordered
• forcing diuresis and altering the patient's urine pH.

PREPARE FOR:

• advanced life support
• intubation and mechanically assisted ventilation
• administration of an antidote based on toxicology screening results
• hemodialysis, peritoneal dialysis, or hemoperfusion.

Nursing Tip

Precaution: If you suspect food poisoning, don't administer antidiarrheals during the first 24 hours after the patient ingests the contaminated food, unless it's absolutely necessary. Diarrhea helps rid the body of the toxin and is a natural response to poisoning.

NONTRAUMATIC EMERGENCIES

National Poison Center Network®
Poison Treatment Chart

How to use this chart:
Locate the substance that has poisoned your patient on the following pages. The number listed after the poison corresponds with the appropriate treatment in the management column below.

Suggested general treatment for poisoning management:

1. There should be no problem in small amounts. **No treatment necessary.** Fluids may be given.

2. Induce vomiting. Give ipecac syrup in the following dosages:
    Under one year of age:
    Two teaspoons followed by at least 2 to 3 glasses of liquid.
    One year and over:
    Give one tablespoon followed by at least 2 to 3 glasses of liquid.
    Do not induce vomiting if the patient is semicomatose, comatose, or convulsing.
    Call Poison Center for additional information.

3. Dilute or neutralize with water or milk. **Do not induce vomiting.** Gastric lavage is indicated. Call Poison Center for specific instructions.

4. Treat symptomatically unless botulism is suspected. Call Poison Center for specific information regarding botulism.

5. Dilute or neutralize with water or milk. **Do not induce vomiting.** Gastric lavage should be avoided. This substance may cause burns of the mucous membranes. Consult EENT specialist following emergency treatment. Call Poison Center for specific information.

6. Immediately wash skin thoroughly with running water. Call Poison Center for further treatment.

7. Immediately wash eyes with a gentle stream of running water. Continue for 15 minutes. Call Poison Center for further treatment.

Continued

National Poison Center Network®
Poison Treatment Chart *Continued*

8. Specific antagonist may be indicated. Call Poison Center.
9. Remove to fresh air. Support respirations. Call Poison Center for further treatment.
10. Call Poison Center for specific instructions.
11. Symptomatic and supportive treatment. **Do not induce vomiting** for ingestions. I.V. naloxone hydrochloride (Narcan) to be given as indicated for respiratory depression.
    Dosage:
    Adult — 0.4 mg I.V.
      May be repeated at 2 to 3 min. intervals.
    Child — 0.01 mg/kg I.V.
      May be repeated at 5 to 10 min. intervals.

NONTRAUMATIC EMERGENCIES

National Poison Center Network®
Poison Treatment Chart *Continued*

A

Antihistamines 2,8
Antiseptics 2
Ant Trap: Kepone Type 1
       Others 2
Aquarium Products 1
Arsenic 2,8
Aspirin 2

B

Baby Oil 1
Ball Point Ink 1
Barbiturates
  Long Acting 2
  Short Acting 10
Bathroom Bowl Cleaner
  Eye Contamination 7
  Ingestion 5
  Inhalation if mixed with
    bleach 9
  Topical 6
Batteries
  Dry Cell (Flashlight). 1
  Mercury (Hearing Aid) 2
  Wet Cell (Automobile) 5
Benzene
  Ingestion 10
  Inhalation 9
  Topical 6
Birth Control Pills 1
Bleaches
  Eye Contamination 7
  Inhalation when mixed
    with acids or alkalies 9
  Liquid Ingestion 1
  Solid Ingestion 5
Boric Acid 2

Bromides 2
Bubble Bath 1
C
Camphor 2
Candles 1
Caps
  Less than One Roll 1
  More than One Roll 2
Carbon Monoxide 9
Carbon Tetrachloride
  Ingestion 2
  Inhalation 9
  Topical 6
Chalk .1
Chlorine Bleach
          . . . . .See Bleaches
Cigarettes
  Less than One 1
  One or More 2
Clay 1
Cleaning Fluids 10
Cleanser (household) 1
Clinitest Tablets 5
Cold Remedies 10
Cologne
  Less than 15 cc 1
  More than 15 cc 2
Contraceptive Pills 1
Corn-Wart Removers 5
Cosmetics
        . . . . See Specific Type
Cough Medicines 10
Crayons
  Children's 1
  Others 2
Cyanide 8
Continued

National Poison Center Network®
Poison Treatment Chart *Continued*

D

Dandruff Shampoo 2
Dehumidifying Packets 1
Denture Adhesives 1
Denture Cleansers 5
Deodorants
    All Types 1
Deodorizer Cakes 2
Deodorizers, Room 10
Desiccants 1
Detergents
    Electric Dishwasher and
        Phosphate-Free 5
    Liquid-Powder
        (General) 1
Diaper Rash Ointment 1
Dishwasher Detergents
           See Detergents
Disinfectants 3
Drain Cleaners . . . . See Lye
Dyes
    Aniline . . . . . . See Aniline Dyes
    Others 2

E

Electric Dishwasher
    Detergent . . . . See Detergents
Epoxy Glue
    Catalyst 5
    Resin or When Mixed 10
Epsom Salts 2
Ethyl Alcohol . . . . . . See Alcohol
Ethylene Glycol . . See Antifreeze
Eye Makeup 1

F

Fabric Softeners 2

Fertilizers 10
Fish Bowl Additives 1
Food Poisoning 4
Furniture Polish 10

G

Gas (Natural) 9
Gasoline 10
Glue 10
Gun Products 10

H

Hair Dyes
    Eye Contamination 7
    Ingestion 3
    Topical 6
Hallucinogens 5,8
Hand Cream 1
Hand Lotions 1
Herbicides 10
Heroin 8,11
Hormones 1
Hydrochloric Acid . . . . See Acids

I

Inks
    Ballpoint pen 1
    Indelible 2
    Laundry-Marking 2
    Printer's 2
Insecticides
    Ingestion 8
    Topical 6,8
Iodine 5,8
Iron 10
Isopropyl Alcohol . . . See Alcohol

Continued

NONTRAUMATIC
EMERGENCIES

National Poison Center Network®
Poison Treatment Chart *Continued*

Continued

NONTRAUMATIC EMERGENCIES

National Poison Center Network®
Poison Treatment Chart *Continued*

NONTRAUMATIC EMERGENCIES

INDEX

INDEX

INDEX

INDEX